Moral Threats and Dangerous Desires

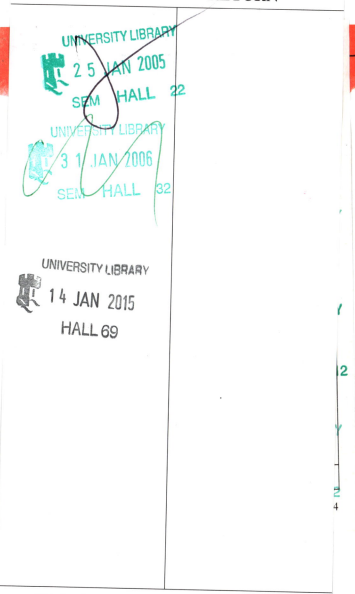

Social Aspects of AIDS

Series Editor: Peter Aggleton
Goldsmiths' College, University of London

Moral Threats and Dangerous Desires:
AIDS in the News Media

Deborah Lupton

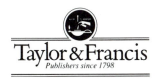

Taylor & Francis
Publishers since 1798

UK   Taylor & Francis Ltd, 4 John St., London WC1N 2ET
USA   Taylor & Francis Inc., 1900 Frost Road, Suite 101, Bristol, PA 19007

First published 1994

A Catalogue Record for this book is available from the British Library

ISBN 0 7484 0179 2
ISBN 0 7484 0180 6 (pbk)

10 0 0525391

Library of Congress Cataloging-in-Publication Data are available on request

Cover design by Barking Dog Art.
Illustration by Hybert • Design & Type
Typeset in 11/13pt Baskerville
by Graphicraft Typesetters Ltd., Hong Kong

Printed in Great Britain by Burgess Science Press, Basingstoke on paper which has a specified pH value on final paper manufacture of not less than 7.5 and is therefore 'acid free'.

Contents

Contents

List of figures

Acknowledgments

Thanks are due to the AIDS Council of New South Wales for providing access to their news clippings files, Simon Chapman and Cathy Waldby, who made helpful comments on parts of the early manuscript, and above all to Peter Aggleton for his detailed editorial criticism. I also thank Gamini Colless for his ongoing support.

The publishers of the following articles gave their permission to reproduce copyright material.

- Apocalypse to banality: changes in metaphors about AIDS in the Australian press, *Australian Journal of Communication*, **18**, 2, pp. 66–74. School of Communication and Organizational Studies, Queensland University of Technology, 1992.
- From complacency to panic: AIDS and heterosexuals in the Australian press, July 1986 to June 1988, *Health Education Research: Theory and Practice*, **7**, 1, pp. 9–20. OUP, 1992.
- Back to complacency: AIDS in the Australian press, March-September 1990, *Health Education Research: Theory and Practice*, **8**, 1, pp. 5–17. OUP, 1993 (co-authored with S. Chapman and W.L. Wong).
- AIDS risk and heterosexuality in the Australian press, *Discourse and Society*, **4**, 3, pp. 307–328. Sage Publications, 1993.
- The condom in the age of AIDS: Newly respectable or still a dirty word? A discourse analysis (in press), *Qualitative Health Research*. Sage Publications.

Series editor's preface

In countries all over the world, the mass media has had a key role to play in constructing public understandings of HIV and AIDS. In perhaps the majority of instances, HIV-related disease has been presented as a condition affecting social and/or demographic minorities – groups whose 'exceptional' behaviour has put them at special risk. Yet at the same time, HIV and AIDS are said to threaten us all: be we heterosexual, lesbian or gay; be we young or somewhat older; be we of minority or majority ethnic status. How does the media manage tensions between these two apparently contradicting stances? How do media messages about the epidemic change over time? How are older health discourses about contagion, plague and death taken up and used in contemporary AIDS reporting? These and other issues are examined here in an empirical study of the ways in which HIV disease, and the communities and individuals affected, have been portrayed in the Australian news media.

Peter Aggleton

Introduction

The Acquired Immunodeficiency Syndrome (AIDS)[1] was unheard of until 1981 but has had an enormous impact upon the popular imagination. Few other diseases this century have been greeted with quite the same degree of fear, loathing, and prejudice against those who develop it. Few other diseases have been the subject of scholarly conferences, meetings, research projects and analysis in such an intensive way. This book employs the methods and theoretical orientation of cultural and media studies to analyse the manner in which AIDS has been constructed in the mass media. The central premise of the book is that the critical cultural examination of news media accounts of AIDS is one way of understanding the disease as a sociocultural phenomenon, that is, as a phenomenon which is not simply a collection of physical symptoms but which is redolent with cultural meaning. The analysis centres on a particular genre of mass media texts: newspaper reporting of AIDS.

The reasons for writing this book generated from an awareness that mainstream public health methods of investigating lay health-related knowledges offered limited understanding of the cultural context in which such knowledges were generated and expressed. One major concern was that public health researchers and practitioners have tended to neglect the importance of the role played by the entertainment and news media in framing public health issues and setting the agenda for policy making and public discussion. Given that the project of health promotion has been defined as to 'enabl[e] people to increase control over, and to improve, their health' (World Health Organization, 1986), the activities and scholarship of this field could potentially include cultural and media studies as integral perspectives in the quest to understand the social context of medicine, health, illness and disease. However, although health promotion incorporates a focus on the communication of information in the health care setting, it is largely neglectful of the cultural and media studies perspectives, despite their growing predominance in communication studies in Australia, Britain, Europe and the United States of America.

The term 'culture' as used by cultural studies scholars is understood both as a way of life including ideas, beliefs, language, institutions and structures of power, and as a range of cultural practices, encompassing artistic forms, architecture, mass produced commodities, everyday activities, eating habits, and media products (Nelson, Treichler and Grossberg, 1992: 5). Using this definition, bodily states and experiences such as illness and disease may be viewed as part of culture. Hence, the agenda for those interested in the communication of messages about health, risk and illness to the general public should include action to understand the types of messages and meanings which are present almost by default in the entertainment and news media in their quest to attract audiences.

However the models of behaviour and knowledge formation which currently underlie health promotion scholarship and activities tend to emphasize rational decision making. As a result, great emphasis is placed upon disseminating information on health risks, on the assumption that this will increase knowledge which in turn will influence people's health protective behaviour. It is generally accepted that health promoters should therefore seek to use the persuasive and saturation power of the mass media to disseminate health-promoting messages. The impact of mass media is most commonly evaluated by quantitatively measuring discrete changes in knowledge, attitudes and behaviours, in a 'before' and 'after' format such as is used in clinical trials of new drugs. This linear approach to communication, privileging 'rationality', rarely recognizes that health knowledges and behaviours are complex social phenomena which have developed over the course of an individual's lifetime as part of everyday activities, are invested with meaning and make very good sense to the individual. Furthermore it is seldom realized that those choices which are deemed 'healthy' by public health bodies are not themselves neutral, but are influenced by ideologies and political concerns.

There is a need for more interpretive social theory and qualitative methods to be applied to issues surrounding sexuality, HIV and AIDS. Qualitative research methods like critical discourse analysis have yet to gain full acceptance in the public health field because they are deemed soft and subjective and do not conform to the 'scientific' methodologies of biomedicine. However, it may be argued that qualitative research is better able to identify the socio-cultural processes that underlie attitudes and behaviour and decision making, and serves to further develop a detailed understanding of the lay beliefs that influence responses to health threats such as AIDS.

Qualitative data collection enabling 'thick' description of a small number of case studies allows researchers to move between public discourses and private practices, exploring the connections between individuals' personal experiences and their understanding of wider issues such as illness, sexuality, morality and death. Such work points the way towards further research which can elucidate the interpersonal aspects of knowledge formation, the findings of which are integral to understanding wider patterns of attitudes and behaviour, explaining how people make sense of their own worlds and give meaning to the practices they engage in during the course of their everyday lives. For example, in Australia, recent AIDS-related qualitative research conducted by Kippax, Crawford, Waldby *et al.* (1990) used individuals' memories about sexual encounters as the basis for discussing popular sayings, beliefs, contradictions, cultural imperatives and metaphors surrounding the negotiation of sexual practices between men and women. They identified some possible reasons for women's inability to negotiate sexual encounters and safer sex with their male partners: in other words, the barriers to implementing 'correct' attitudes. Women were shown to be largely powerless in the heterosexual encounter; sexual practice was not deemed suitable for negotiation because of the taken-for-granted nature of heterosexual sexuality which defines such sexual encounters as 'natural' and therefore needing no discussion. Earlier work (Warwick, Aggleton and Homans, 1988) involving in-depth interviews with British youths identified lay notions that contracting HIV is largely a matter of bad luck (serendipitous logic), and that the virus is easily transmitted (miasmic beliefs). Beliefs emphasized the endogenous (caused by an individual's personal qualities) nature of HIV infection, explaining the common distinctions drawn between 'innocent' and 'guilty' people living with AIDS. Recent in-depth interviews with young university students in Canada found that the respondents, while afraid of contracting HIV, viewed AIDS in the context of other fatal disasters which were unlikely to happen to them, and also held out hopes of a cure, reasoning that even if they did become infected, there would be a cure in time. In addition, AIDS was viewed as being caused by certain individuals who engaged in particular types of sexual activities, rather than a virus, and the respondents distanced themselves from such individuals, placing importance on selecting the 'right' type of sexual partner (Maticka-Tyndale, 1992).

When such deep-seated, almost subconscious, beliefs pertaining to AIDS, sexuality and health issues are identified, the question is begged, 'How were these beliefs constructed?'. Given the pervasiveness and popularity of the entertainment and news mass media, it is inevitable that they, in concert with formal health education programmes, interpersonal communication and personal experiences, are influential in the development and subsequent shaping of lay health beliefs. In the case of AIDS, the popular media, especially the news media, have played an extremely important role in drawing upon pre-established knowledge and belief systems to create this new disease as a meaningful phenomenon, particularly in regions dominated by the mass media such as westernized countries. From the time that the symptoms of AIDS were first recorded, in the absence of other sources of easily accessible information, the news media have defined AIDS for the developed world, set the agenda for public discussion of AIDS issues, and influenced key decisions of policy makers. For these reasons, a critical examination of the representation of AIDS in the popular media, as well as research investigating the response of audiences to the messages and meanings disseminated in the media, are of major importance in understanding the construction of AIDS-related knowledges, or the epistemology of AIDS. However, few scholars have attempted a thorough, detailed textual and historical analysis of the ways in which news accounts of AIDS have been constructed and have changed over the decade and more in which AIDS has been known.

Moving away from didacticism and the reliance upon simplistic social psychological models of behaviour and quantitative understandings of the creation of meaning in mass media products, this book adopts a social constructionist approach to the analysis of AIDS as news as a cultural phenomenon. The social constructionist approach as applied to understanding the social aspects of medicine, health and disease derives from philosophical and sociological inquiries into the social construction of knowledge, or 'ways of knowing' (Berger and Luckmann, 1967). Social constructionism takes a relativist perspective, viewing knowledges, including those under the rubric of science and medicine, as being dynamic, firmly embedded in, and influenced by, their historical and political settings. While diseases, symptoms or illnesses are not regarded as 'imaginary', the ways in which they are described, experienced and treated by medicine and by the lay public are regarded as social products which are transitory rather than fixed (Wright and Treacher, 1982; Nicolson and McLaughlin, 1987; Brandt, 1991). The constructionist perspective recognizes that diseases thereby become meaningful; their meanings may be used to impute blame, to allow moral judgements to be expressed, to obscure patriarchy and paternalism, to maintain powerful interests, and to exert control.

An examination of the language and discourses used to describe and account for health, illness and disease is vital to the constructionist project, for it is acknowledged that linguistic and discursive processes are integral in the determination of subjectivity, making the world intelligible to social actors. Medical and health issues provide sites for discursive battles over meaning, at which debates over power, gender, sexual preference and social class are contested in the public domain. The ways that people learn about and understand a disease or illness, the types of experiences they have when ill, the moral judgements made about the causes of illness, are all mediated by language. Illness is not only physically experienced, but is spoken: words are used in the attempt to convey the pain or discomfort an ill person feels; words direct the relationship between doctor or nurse and patient; words nominate which kinds of people are considered to be 'at risk' of developing an illness and how they should be treated. Language is central to the meaning of illness. Therefore, the analysis of language has the potential to demonstrate 'the process by which biology and culture interact' (Brandt, 1988a: 417) in the social construction of disease, and the ways in which western culture uses disease to define social boundaries.

By using textual analysis to analyse press representations of AIDS over time, insight may be provided into some of the dominant beliefs, values and anxieties extant in a society not only about AIDS but about broader socio-cultural notions concerning disease, illness and health risks. Such an approach is likely to offer more illuminating explanations of societies' and individuals' responses to AIDS than the traditional insistence upon the quantification of media messages into rigid content categories, and controlled laboratory-based evaluations of media effects. It offers particular insights into the socio-cultural context in which attitudes toward people with HIV or AIDS and people's perceptions of risk from HIV infection are developed and the responses of governments to the AIDS epidemic are formulated.

This book is interdisciplinary: the perspectives of the history of medicine, textual analysis, media and cultural studies, medical anthropology and the sociology of health and illness all find some expression within. For comparison purposes, Chapter One reviews relevant, previously published, studies of news media's coverage of AIDS in various countries, discussing how critical analysis has been used as an effective strategy of cultural activism. Chapter Two provides a more detailed methodological background of media analysis. It looks at the elements integral to the construction and production of news texts and outlines the methods of critical discourse analysis used in the analysis presented here. The next three chapters describe the findings of an in-depth study of AIDS reporting in the Australian press. As AIDS reporting now spans over ten years and many thousands of news texts, analysis has been confined to specific periods of reporting. Chapter Three covers the early years of AIDS reporting (1981 to 1985), while Chapter Four centres around the two year period between July 1986 and June 1988, during which the pivotal 'Grim Reaper' AIDS education campaign, used by the Australian government to raise awareness of AIDS and warn all sectors of society (including heterosexuals) that they may be at risk of contracting HIV, was released. Due to its controversial and shocking nature, the campaign inspired massive mass media coverage of AIDS issues. Chapter Five discusses AIDS reporting during a seven-month period in 1990, and ends with general conclusions. Chapter Six moves from a micro- to a macro-focus, placing the news texts in their broader social, historical and political contexts, with detailed discussion of the regulation of dangerous sexual desires, deviance and the 'other', gender politics, body boundaries and the fear of invasion, and discourses on risk and morality. The Epilogue brings the analysis into the early 1990s, making observations and predictions about AIDS as news into the second decade and beyond, and focusing upon the role played by well-known people in shaping public debates on AIDS.

While the explicit focus of the analysis of newspaper reports is upon those published in Australia, the detailed discussion of the historical and cultural factors bringing to bear upon discourses on AIDS in the Australian press makes constant reference to broad social trends that have affected the western world as a whole. As such, the book serves several functions which have wider concerns than AIDS, including illuminating the role played by discursive processes in the interaction between the western model of medicine, notions of disease causation, public health policy and everyday knowledges about health and disease, and demonstrating the advocacy potential of critical discourse analysis to inform political activism and resistance.

Notes

1 For brevity's sake, the word AIDS is used throughout this book as shorthand for the more encompassing term HIV/AIDS, except where this usage would cause

confusion or is strictly incorrect. For example, individuals are described as HIV antibody positive rather than AIDS positive when they have not developed any of the symptoms of AIDS but have antibodies for the Human Immunodeficiency Virus. Similarly, the test measuring antibodies to HIV is referred to throughout as an HIV antibody test, not the incorrect term 'AIDS test'. However, direct quotations from news texts retain the original terminology.

Chapter 1

AIDS as News

AIDS was first reported to the world in 1981 when five cases of *Pneumocystis carinii* pneumonia and 26 cases of the hitherto rare cancer *Kaposi's sarcoma*, associated with extreme immune deficiency, were reported among young gay men in the USA. By 1982 several articles had been published in American medical journals concerning this mystifying new disease, which already was being described as a 'serious public health problem' by virtue of its high mortality rate among young, previously healthy individuals (CDC Taskforce, 1982: 252). In late 1982, when the tally of cases identified worldwide was 788 (Waterson, 1983: 745), medical journal articles began referring to the condition as the Acquired Immunodeficiency Syndrome or its acronym, AIDS. It was during this early discovery phase that AIDS was labelled a 'Gay Plague' in the medical literature. Most articles published in medical journals describing the disease included in their title a reference to gay men, despite evidence that women and heterosexual men were susceptible to the disease. Other high risk groups in the USA, including injecting drug users, people with haemophilia, and Haitians were also largely disregarded, as the attention of researchers became more and more centred upon gay men with AIDS.

There is no doubt that in the short space of time AIDS has been 'known' in the western world, it has commanded a huge media interest. In 1985 the American news story wire service United Press International reported that AIDS was one of the top four news-making issues, while the Associated Press placed it fifth and Encyclopaedia Britannica rated it sixth on a worldwide basis. In 1986 these sources all ranked AIDS ninth in international news value (Hughey, Norton and Sullivan-Norton, 1989: 56–7). In the quest for profit, newspapers and magazines must try to maximize their readership. Their agenda is not explicitly to disseminate health information *per se*, but to entertain.

Hence, they focus upon drama, controversy, human interest, brevity and simplicity in news stories. Hence too, AIDS has received enormous coverage in the popular media. The news media's desire to publish sensational and unusual stories to attract consumers' attention was fulfilled by the association of AIDS with male homosexuality, heterosexual promiscuity, prostitution and injecting drug use: all behaviours which inspire prurience and voyeurism. All of the necessary conditions for 'good' news were thus provided by this new disease, and assisted in making AIDS – at least at first – a media sensation.

The ways in which the phenomenon of AIDS has been represented in the entertainment and news mass media have played an important role in the development of shared cultural meanings about AIDS. Weber and Goldmeier (1983) wrote a case note for the *British Medical Journal* about the hundreds of patients they had recently seen with anxiety about AIDS, of which three had severe psychiatric illness with fear of AIDS as the dominant feature. One man had watched a television documentary on AIDS in April 1983, following which he had developed an irrational conviction that he was incubating AIDS, suicidal thoughts and fear of contaminating others. A second patient complained of acute depression, malaise, night sweats and impairment of concentration. These symptoms had begun when he had read a newspaper article on AIDS. The third patient had seen the documentary also, which he watched on video over 30 times. He developed intense anxiety about AIDS, was unable to work and contemplated suicide. The authors believe that 'in each case the condition was precipitated by particular media coverage of the AIDS epidemic' (Weber and Goldmeier, 1983: 420).

These individuals represent extreme cases of reaction to mass media news coverage of AIDS and it is unlikely that many others in the general public have been so affected. However, it has often been speculated that the news media have had an impact upon everyday and popular beliefs about AIDS. The importance of the mass media, most particularly television, newspapers and magazines, as major sources for individuals in western countries for information about AIDS, whether it be accurate or distorted, has emerged in many large scale studies of AIDS-related knowledge, attitudes, beliefs and behaviour carried out in a number of countries (Ross and Carson, 1988; White, Phillips, Pitts *et al.*, 1988; Dolan, Corber and Zacour, 1990; Carducci, Frasca, Matteelli *et al.*, 1990; Herlitz and Brorsson, 1990; Abraham, Sheeran, Abrams *et al.*, 1991). One Australian study (Bray and Chapman, 1991) conducted two randomized telephone surveys of Sydney adults in 1988 and 1989 in which a total of 1352 interviewees were asked to recall, without prompting, any AIDS programmes, articles or advertisements in the print or electronic media; 92 per cent in 1988, and 93 per cent in 1989, could recall at least one advertisement or programme about AIDS on television. While only a minority of interviewees could recall a radio programme or advertisement, approximately half of them recalled articles about AIDS in newspapers or magazines. Those most often recalled were the individual stories of real people whose lives had been affected by AIDS.

It has also been asserted that individuals perceived to be at high risk from HIV infection, or those identified as seropositive, may be psychologically adversely affected by homophobic statements made in the media, or by statements that assume that HIV seropositivity is an inevitable death sentence (M.W. Ross, 1989: 79). Pictorial representations of people (most usually gay men) living with AIDS in the popular media have routinely depicted them as emaciated, disfigured, ashamed, despairing and lacking hope (Crimp, 1992). In response to these images and representations at least one HIV antibody positive man has publicly commented that:

> People with HIV disease, and especially people with AIDS, are constantly reminded that they are probably going to die. You turn on the television or open a newspaper and, in the context of an item of AIDS, you will see yourself described in terms which make it clear that, in society's eyes, you are finished.
>
> Grimshaw, 1987: 256

While quantitative studies routinely refer to the 'mass media' as an important source of AIDS information, little attention has been paid by public health researchers to singling out the relative importance of unplanned messages and meanings about AIDS issues disseminated in the entertainment and news media which compete for audiences' attention with planned education campaigns. Few researchers have specifically attempted to determine the reaction of audiences to the entertainment mass media's representation of AIDS using small-scale qualitative methods. However audience response research undertaken by Tulloch (1989) investigated the response of the audience to the episode of the Australian television series *A Country Practice* which depicted the fictionalized story of a young girl who contracts HIV after sharing needles. Small groups of students (178 in all) were shown the episode at school, and were taped talking (without a teacher or researcher present) about the key messages in the text. Tulloch found that the episode had a significant effect on the students' awareness of needle sharing as a high priority risk behaviour for HIV infection. Many of them mentioned this risk behaviour for the first time after seeing the episode. Additionally, the discussion of the students revealed that they made sense of the episode according to understandings of drug use current within the particular subculture to which they belonged. Tulloch (1989: 123) concludes that 'the transmission of health messages is a process of negotiation between several different cultures'. In a later paper (1992), he notes that a larger group of students shown the episode lacked identification with the characters and the AIDS education message, even though the intention of the producers of the episode was to generalize the risk of AIDS.

In another study, Kitzinger and colleagues (Kitzinger, 1990; Kitzinger and Miller, 1991) utilized several methods of researching the influence of the British news media in shaping the beliefs of the general public about AIDS. The researchers were particularly interested in how members of the audience interpret what they hear and see in the news media. Kitzinger and colleagues worked with pre-existing groups of people from a wide range of socio-economic backgrounds resident in Scotland. Study participants were invited to engage in such exercises as 'The News Game', in which they were asked to play the role of journalist in producing a news story related to a set of pictures, thereby initiating discussion about AIDS and the media, particularly concerning the value judgements, information and narrative structures apparent in the media. One major finding was that the participants' most popular belief about the origins of AIDS was that it came from Africa. According to the participants, their primary source of information was the news media. Many participants specifically recalled the ways in which early reporting of AIDS linked it to Africa, Haiti or the Third World. The researchers found striking similarities between audience understandings of 'African AIDS' and news reports. Kitzinger and Miller (1991: 20) concluded that journalists both drew upon and helped to reproduce certain cultural assumptions about AIDS and Africans in their reports. These assumptions were then reflected in the respondents' attitudes to AIDS.

The conclusions drawn by researchers engaged in this type of audience response research have therefore suggested that the tenor of coverage of AIDS issues in such popular media products as soap operas and news reports may be very influential in the construction of lay health beliefs and knowledges relating to AIDS. Yet such findings also demonstrate that audiences respond to media products in complex and sometimes unexpected ways, and are not simply passive receptacles for the preferred meanings of the producers.

AIDS in the news media

To add a further dimension to audience response research, it is necessary to document in detail the types of information, messages, meanings and discourses present in such media. There has been very little analysis published which has attempted to go beyond the surface meaning of reportage of medicine, health, illness and disease. One exception is the AIDS epidemic, which has sparked a plethora of creative, critical and insightful responses from media analysts, many of whom centre their attention upon the ways in which the disease has been depicted in the news. As one of the progenitors of cultural studies, Stuart Hall, recently remarked, the advent of AIDS has inspired the field of cultural studies to analyse 'the constitutive and political nature of representation itself, about its complexities, about the effects of language, about textuality as a site of life and death' (Hall, 1992: 285).

The vast majority of large-scale research into the media coverage of AIDS has been undertaken of the news media in the USA (Albert, 1986a, 1986b; Baker, 1986; Hughey, Norton and Sullivan-Norton, 1989; King, 1990; Austin, 1990; Clarke, 1991, 1992; Nelkin, 1991; Rogers, Dearing and Chang, 1991; Colby and Cook, 1991) and the UK (Wellings, 1988; Murray, 1991; Beharrell, 1991, 1993; Berridge, 1991), but the news media in France (Herzlich and Pierret, 1989), Puerto Rico (Cunningham, 1989), West Germany (Jones, 1992) and Canada (Clarke, 1991) have also been examined. Others have taken a comparative approach, contrasting news coverage of AIDS in San Francisco and London (Temoshok, Grade and Zich, 1989), Japan and the USA (Dearing, 1992) and a number of European countries (Grube and Boehme-Duerr, 1988). These findings are extremely useful in providing information about the broad patterns of AIDS reporting in the overseas news media. Because of their generally systematic approach, the findings from many such analyses may be generalized to a large body of news media.

Several studies of AIDS as news have shown that there have been important changes in the focus of the coverage over time. Following initial phases of panic reporting and dramatic headlines, AIDS news coverage in western countries by the late 1980s appeared to have been rendered routine, largely losing its dramatic qualities. Herzlich and Pierret (1989) identified four main phases in the French reporting of AIDS. The first they entitled 'The mysterious illness', and place between January 1982 and April 1983. During that time, AIDS was first mentioned in the press and underwent a 'naming process'. Press reports focused upon quantitative data which stated the actual or projected number of cases nationally and worldwide, and concern was expressed about the rapid spread of AIDS. AIDS was perceived in two paradoxical ways: one perception related to its 'accidental' nature, the other to its potential to cause a worldwide catastrophe. It was presented as an emergency, about which 'something must be done'.

Herzlich and Pierret named the second phase in French reporting 'The construction of a "social phenomenon"'. This phase, spanning May 1983 to May 1984, was bounded by two scientific events: the publication of a report in the medical journal *Science* about the viral origin of AIDS, and the official announcement by American authorities of the discovery of the virus that probably caused AIDS. During this time, the number of articles in the French daily newspapers increased tenfold. According to Herzlich and Pierret (1989: 1237), it was during this phase that the 'AIDS social phenomenon' was 'constructed scientifically, economically, morally, and culturally'. AIDS had become more than a serious illness: it had become a public issue. In French newspapers the topic of the year in 1983 was AIDS. This period of intense press interest was followed by a phase the authors called 'A relative calm', lasting from June 1984 to March 1985, in which fewer articles about AIDS were published. Articles during this time mainly dealt with scientific issues and the spread of AIDS to other countries and groups. Between April 1985 and June 1986, press interest in AIDS revived, and this phase Herzlich and Pierret accordingly titled 'Gaining momentum'. During this time the first international conference on AIDS was held, the dispute over the identification of the virus had flared up again, a debate about the systematic testing of blood donors occurred, AIDS was appearing in prisons and political interventions in the spread of the disease were becoming explicit. AIDS was no longer a problem of individuals alone, but now was a problem for the government. In addition, Herzlich and Pierret assert, AIDS had by then been fully constructed as a social phenomenon; it was no longer presented as mysterious or novel.

Three peaks in American news coverage between June 1981 and December 1988 can be identified: May 1983, July 1985 and February 1987 (Rogers, Dearing and Chang, 1991). AIDS was initially ignored by the mainstream American news media, which were uncomfortable discussing homosexuality, fearing a negative response from audiences, and which did not consider the disease newsworthy enough while it seemed confined to the gay population. In 1982, for example, although by then there had been 800 reported cases and 350 deaths from AIDS in the USA, there were only six stories about AIDS on the major network news, and few articles appeared in newspapers and magazines (Nelkin, 1991; Cook and Colby, 1992). Indeed, for five years into the AIDS epidemic, the influential *New York Times* refused to use the word 'gay' except within quoted passages (Rogers, Dearing and Chang, 1991). In May 1983, the rise in news coverage followed the publication of an editorial in the *Journal of the American Medical Association* concerning the possibility of AIDS being 'transmitted' through everyday close contact, but interest subsequently declined.

An analysis of all AIDS-related articles which appeared in American national circulation magazines between May 1982 and December 1983 found that people living with AIDS, especially gay men, were portrayed in magazines as 'experiencing a reign of terror justified by an exponentially increasing death toll' (Albert, 1986a: 170). Gay men were represented as reaping the rewards of their 'depravity', and there was an implicit use of blame as an indicator of social worth. AIDS was thus presented as a problem which affected only a small and deviant group of people. When Rock Hudson's illness from AIDS was announced in July 1985, there was a dramatic increase in news stories about AIDS in the American media lasting until his death in October, which continued until December that same year with coverage of a boy with HIV infection, Ryan White, and the discrimination he faced in connection with school attendance (Rogers, Dearing and Chang, 1991; Nelkin, 1991; Cook and Colby, 1992). The importance of AIDS as a rapidly growing epidemic was reinforced by *Time* magazine's publication of a cover story in August 1985 with the headline

AIDS, THE GROWING THREAT: WHAT'S BEING DONE.

The American news media's attention dropped again during 1986, but rose to a new height in early 1987 with increasing attention on mandatory testing and privacy issues, the heterosexual transmission of HIV, and Presidents Reagan and Bush's first public statements on AIDS (Rogers, Dearing and Chang, 1991; Cook and Colby, 1992). In February 1987 *Time* magazine again published a cover story on AIDS, this time focusing on the threat posed to heterosexuals:

THE BIG CHILL: HOW HETEROSEXUALS ARE COPING WITH AIDS

Testing and privacy issues dominated press coverage in the late 1980s; by then the annual International AIDS Conference in June provided the annual peak of coverage in the American news media (Colby and Cook, 1991).

Berridge (1991) asserts that British media coverage, particularly that of the press, appeared broadly to parallel the chronology of policy development. She identified four stages of reporting: 1981–3; 1983–5; 1986–7; and from 1988 onwards. In concert with other commentators, e.g. Watney (1987) and Wellings (1988), she notes the dominance of the 'gay plague' representation of AIDS in the earliest stage of British reporting. However, she suggests that from mid-1983 the focus shifted to questions about the safety of the blood supply and heterosexual transmission in Africa, the latter topic raising the spectre of a possible heterosexual epidemic in Britain. The issues of AIDS in prisons and the death of Rock Hudson dominated coverage in 1985. In 1986 the focus of policy changed again as the key issue became the national emergency posed by the disease to the entire British population. Berridge identifies qualitative differences between television and press coverage of AIDS during this period: according to her, the emphasis of television news coverage was upon minimizing the threat posed by AIDS to the general population using liberal notions of education, while the press adopted a New Right agenda favouring testing and quarantine.

The question of the risk posed by AIDS to heterosexuals was a major issue in British media reporting during 1988–90 (Murray, 1991; Berridge, 1991; Beharrell, 1991). British news accounts were characterized by a heated debate concerning whether or not heterosexuals were at risk from AIDS following a government-sponsored campaign directed at heterosexuals in February 1988. During this period, the tabloid press in particular promoted the view that heterosexual risk had been much exaggerated and alleged that 'guilty' AIDS patients were consuming more than their fair share of resources (Murray, 1991: 39). The liberal, 'quality' press were more likely to emphasize heterosexual risk and be supportive of the government's attempts to educate the general public, while the conservative press, both broadsheet and tabloid, was far more negative and critical of the education efforts: 'often, health education [was] depicted as at best a waste of time and money, at worst a sinister conspiracy' (Beharrell, 1991: 27).

After 1988, Berridge notes a normalization of AIDS in both British government policy and news media coverage. In this most recent period, she identifies a decline in the intensity of media coverage, accompanied by claims about the 'myth of heterosexual spread'. One news editor was quoted by Berridge (1991: 181) as stating in late 1989 that AIDS has become 'a boring story . . . The only stories now would be a miracle cure or a massive rise in heterosexual spread – AIDS is a buried subject'. 'Gay Plague' representations of AIDS were therefore, according to Berridge (1991: 181) 'a response which was both historically and media specific'. She asserts that the diminishing of such representations in favour of a normalization of AIDS has resulted in the news coverage of gay people living with AIDS being vastly reduced.

In most western countries, well-known 'news actors' and 'news sources' have influenced the agenda for discussion of AIDS issues. In the British news media, for example, conservative news sources and news actors such as members of parliament were privileged over more radical individuals or groups, such as feminist and gay activists. One notable example of the publicizing of this conservative view occurred in November 1989, when a member of the British All Party Parliamentary Group on AIDS, Lord Kilbracken, claimed that there was only one proven British case of AIDS attributable to heterosexual transmission, and that therefore government agencies were over-emphasizing the AIDS risk faced by heterosexuals. Kilbracken's standing in the community as a prominent politician gave a discourse emphasizing the 'myth of heterosexual AIDS' an opportunity to enter wider circulation via the British news media (Beharrell, 1993).

An analysis of AIDS discourse in two West German news magazines (*Der Spiegel* and *Stern*) (Jones, 1992) noted that the magazines employed pre-existing discourses about gays, women, injecting drug users, prostitutes, blacks and people with haemophilia, all of whom are minority groups. Jones examined the way in which governmental discourse and journalistic discourse combined to create particular definitions of AIDS and people living with AIDS which were 'ultimately extremely political in intent and effect' (Jones, 1992: 440). Jones' analysis focused upon representations of AIDS between 1986 and 1990, and therefore moves on from discussing the 'gay plague' era of reporting to more recent portrayals of AIDS. Jones identified in the magazine reports a distinction drawn between 'good gays' (those who get tested for HIV, stop having sex of any kind, and co-operate with medical authorities) and 'bad gays' (those who continue to practice unsafe sex). In the West German press, discussion of gay behaviour was superseded in 1987 by concern about the risk posed by prostitutes and injecting drug users as potential links in the 'chain of infection' to the heterosexual population. Prostitutes were depicted as the objectified sources of contagion, while their male customers were 'innocent victims and witnesses to the crime' (Jones, 1992: 446). Injecting drug users were represented as 'a dark, pathological threat' (Jones, 1992: 447). People with haemophilia, although portrayed as innocent victims of HIV infection, were also subject to stigmatization because of the dominant ideology of disease as a failure of the individual. According to Jones, the West German magazine articles emphasized that control was the route to prevention, including self-control over sexuality and state control of marriage, prisons and safer-sex education. Personalized accounts of people who had contracted HIV emphasized that the individual had transgressed in some way.

This analysis points to the ways in which women have been portrayed in news media reports on AIDS. Due mainly to a obsession with male gay sexuality, women, both heterosexual and lesbian, have largely been absent in coverage of AIDS issues. The notable exception, as suggested by Jones, is female prostitutes, who have been routinely represented as a locus of contagion. A study of AIDS reports in the *New York Times* and the *Washington Post* between 1985 and 1988 (King, 1990) similarly found that despite lack of epidemiological evidence demonstrating that they posed a threat to their clients, female prostitutes were represented as vectors of HIV. In most western countries it was not until 1986, in concert with the increasing emphasis on the impact of AIDS upon heterosexuals, that the news media began to discuss the position of women in the epidemic. In her analysis of the portrayal of women in American television AIDS documentaries screened during 1986 and 1987, Juhasz (1990: 27), observes that they were depicted as 'contained threats', allowing them to be positioned simultaneously as 'iconographic site of danger and as easily controlled subject'. There were, however, distinctions made between categories of women: on the one hand, the 'safe' women (middle class, white, married); and on the other, the 'dangerous' women (prostitutes, non-white, working class, single mothers, 'promiscuous'), while lesbians were simply not mentioned. Prostitutes were routinely portrayed as dangerous reservoirs of infection, needful of control, while white, respectable, married women were the 'innocent', acceptable, respected spokeswomen for female people living with AIDS (Juhasz, 1990: 27).

The news media coverage of AIDS has often incorporated elements of racism. According to Hammonds (1986), the African–American press in the USA, and particularly the leading magazines *Ebony* and *Essence*, neglected coverage of AIDS until 1986. Hammonds found that almost all the articles in these magazines that subsequently appeared that year tried to indicate that African–Americans were at risk of infection while also trying to avoid the implication that AIDS is a 'black' disease, thus under-emphasizing the socio-economic context in which HIV is spread. In these magazines, there was a failure to discuss wider policy issues to do with the African–American community, and homosexuality and bisexuality were dealt with very conservatively and pejoratively. The response of the magazines to the racist stereotypes linking blacks, disease and immorality was to argue that blacks should demonstrate their respectability, thereby attempting to fit into dominant white ideologies concerning appropriate behaviour. Hammonds notes that the American mainstream (white) press during the same period was largely silent on the subject of the heterosexual spread of HIV in Africa, and neglected coverage of the risk posed to underprivileged blacks and Hispanics in American cities via injecting drug use, while simultaneously emphasizing the 'new' phenomenon of heterosexual AIDS amongst whites in the USA.

Dada (1990) presented examples of racism in British AIDS reporting. He makes the point that in Britain the plight of blacks and other ethnic minorities at risk from AIDS has been more invisible than that of gay men. Despite this invisibility of British blacks, Dada asserts that the blame for AIDS has often been levelled at African blacks, and believes that the gay community has perpetuated this stereotype in defence. Austin (1990) deconstructed images of AIDS and Africa as presented in popular newspapers and magazines printed in the USA. He argues that the depiction of AIDS in Africa is redolent with racist notions, in which constructions of 'Africa', 'the African', the 'prostitute', and the 'homosexual' are interweaved and linked with historical notions of 'Africa', the black subject, sexuality, and disease in white western imagination. Similarly, in the West German press (Jones, 1992) Africa was depicted as a 'Death House' or the 'land of AIDS', carrying the guilt as the putative source of AIDS.

The AIDS epidemic in the USA has received the attention of the news media in several other countries, both because of the high incidence of the disease in the USA, and that country's elite status. For example, Grube and Bochme-Duerr (1988) analysed all articles about AIDS in issues of five international news magazines published between the third week of September 1985 until the third week of March 1986. They found that there was more news relating to AIDS in the USA than other countries, and even though at that time France had the highest prevalence of AIDS cases of the European countries, it did not receive very high coverage by comparison. An analysis of the Puerto Rican press coverage of AIDS issues between 1982 and 1988 (Cunningham, 1989) noted that the Puerto Rican press was very derivative of that of the USA: more than two thirds of their AIDS articles originated outside Puerto Rico, the majority of them coming from the USA.

Several studies of AIDS as news have found that there is a

symbiotic relationship between press and other news coverage and government policy about AIDS. In Puerto Rico, for example, Cunningham (1989) contends that articles about AIDS printed in the Puerto Rico press were used as a means of contrasting the ideologies of those in power in Puerto Rico rather than communicating information about the disease itself. People with AIDS as individuals were generally rendered invisible in the debate. Those to receive press attention were members of occupational groups or unions who were concerned about the risks of contracting HIV through work practices. For that reason, suggested Cunningham, the general public in Puerto Rico has tended to perceive AIDS as more a political than a medical question. By contrast, in Britain, planned health education messages about AIDS risk conforming to government policy were often contradicted by the information and messages disseminated in news accounts (Wellings, 1988).

Cultural analysis and cultural activism

The AIDS epidemic has inspired a growing number of cultural theorists to analyse in depth the language used to represent disease. AIDS, as lethal, debilitating, stigmatizing and frightening as it is, has proved a powerful catalyst and inspiration for efforts attempting to understand illness and disease as social constructions. As Watney (1989a: 64) has commented; '[i]ndeed, it could be said that contemporary debates in cultural studies, women's studies, psychoanalytic criticism, textual analysis, the theory of ideology, and so on, have been preparing us for a better understanding of what is now being done – and what is not being done – in the name of AIDS'.

In addition to the analyses of AIDS as news reviewed above, there has been a wealth of critical commentary about AIDS discourse in the news media which has been undertaken mainly by British and American scholars. This commentary, originating as it does from the traditions of critical literary and cultural theory, and fuelled by the concerns of radical gay and feminist politics, is not primarily concerned with the systematic enumeration of elements of news coverage of AIDS but with more closely examining the reproduction of power relations and the ideological and political functions of language in news texts. In 1989, commentaries on AIDS as news were published in two important collections of essays. The first volume (*Taking Liberties: AIDS and Cultural Politics*, 1989, edited by Erica Carter and Simon Watney) was based on an innovative conference in London sponsored by the

Institute of Contemporary Arts. The second (*AIDS: Cultural Analysis, Cultural Activism*, 1989b, edited by Douglas Crimp) is a collection of reprinted articles which had originally appeared in a special issue of the literary criticism journal *October*. As the titles of these collections suggest, the main theme of both was the necessity of 'making sense' of the AIDS epidemic in a critical manner, by analysing AIDS discourse, and by using this knowledge to act politically, to resist discriminatory policies and actions against people with AIDS, and at risk from AIDS.

A contributor to both volumes, Simon Watney, has been prolific in publishing work on the cultural politics of AIDS, particularly with respect to the media's portrayal of homosexuality. Watney's reading of media reports of AIDS deconstructs their messages to their psychoanalytic and symbolic level and is activist in that he is at pains to show the discrimination against and the oppression of gay men in press accounts of AIDS. His rhetoric often borders on the polemical but his main points, particularly in his early work, *Policing Desire: Pornography, AIDS and the Media* (Watney, 1987), and a chapter published in the volume edited by Crimp (1989b), were timely, enlightening and well-made. Watney's work has been paralleled by that of other British cultural commentators with similar backgrounds in contemporary arts such as Carter (1989), Williamson (1989) and Marshall (1990). In the USA, Crimp (1989a), Gilman (1989), Treichler (1988, 1989), Patton (1989a, 1989b, 1990) and Grover (1989, 1992a, 1992b) have contributed to the cultural analysis of AIDS as represented in the media. Significantly, few of these commentators are employed academically by an institution with medical affiliations; the majority lecture in the arts and humanities, in areas as diverse as photography, French, linguistics, humane studies, and media/film studies.

Analyses such as these of the AIDS epidemic have often taken an overtly political stance. That is, they emerge from a viewpoint which is seeking to change and to resist, as it dissects AIDS as a social phenomenon. Like members of the feminist movement, AIDS cultural activists have focused their attention upon the mass media as sources of the reproduction of oppressive ideologies. They have addressed the need to identify and attack discriminatory representations of people living with AIDS. Most cultural activists are from the ranks of gay men and women who have seen their friends and lovers die, and who are angry about the continued discrimination, stigma, ignorance and sheer apathy to which gay men with HIV or AIDS have been subjected on the part of government officials, medical practitioners, research scientists and drug companies as well as the mass media. Their critical analyses of representations of AIDS in public forums and the medical literature have contributed to and documented the achievements of gay activists in their attempts to resist limiting and stigmatizing cultural mythologies and imagery; see, for example, the essays and artwork collected in Crimp (1989b) and Boffin and Gupta (1990).

Such 'cultural activism' has demonstrated the value of critical scholarship in informing struggles to resist hegemonic ideologies. AIDS activist groups, by using a sophisticated understanding of the importance of language and visual representations, have comprised one of the most successful community movements to challenge medical dominance and scientific authority, questioning traditional restrictions on access to and control over medico-scientific knowledge and resisting the role of the passive patient or experimental subject (Treichler, 1991).

Summary

It is evident that news coverage of AIDS has shared certain common features in most western countries. These include a general neglect of AIDS while it seemed confined to gay men, contradictory and confusing coverage, the tendency of dramatic news accounts to incite panic, the absence of certain social groups in news accounts and the emphatic presence of others, the ability of prominent people to influence coverage of AIDS regardless of their medical expertise or personal experience, and an emphasis upon personalizing the illness experience. AIDS reporting in western nations has invoked imagery associated with homophobia, fear, violence, contamination, invasion, vilification, racism, sexism, deviance, heroism and xenophobia. As subsequent chapters shall demonstrate, discourses of AIDS in Australian press coverage of the disease have drawn upon similar pre-constructed ideologies and narratives to make sense of this new disease.

Chapter 2

Analysing News

Mass media texts such as television programmes and newspaper articles are important primary sources for cultural and social research. Indeed, it is becoming recognized in all areas of social research that such texts are sensitive barometers of social process and change (Jensen, 1991; Fairclough, 1992). The analysis of these texts has many advantages for scholars who are interested in behaviour and societal attitudes. Such texts, once created, remain unchanging, and available for further analysis. The text may be copied, and used by other scholars, or reanalysed. Mass media texts are therefore ideal for studying long-term changes in attitudes, concerns, ideologies and power relations.

News accounts of health and illness differ from many other popular media texts in that they have the weight of 'expert' opinion, 'reality' and 'fact' behind them. Hence the news media wield a certain power as a lobby group, with the potential to influence government policy. As Nelkin (1987: 82) points out, 'By creating public issues out of events, the press can force regulatory agencies to action simply out of concern for their public image'. News media attention to a health issue can result in funding being made more easily available for research in that area. Even if the results of medical or public health research are inconclusive or barely statistically significant, if they appear in a prestigious journal, have a well-known person as one of the authors, the subject is deemed interesting to the public, or the conclusions made by the authors are provocative, then they will be judged newsworthy (Klaidman, 1990). The choice of language in news accounts is particularly important, for 'selective use of language can trivialize an event or render it important; marginalize some groups, empower others; define an issue as an urgent problem or reduce it to a routine' (Nelkin, 1991: 303).

In health research, the methodology used to document media representations has generally adopted a quantitative approach which reduces media content to relatively simple messages which can be enumerated. Quantitative content analysis involves the systematic quantification of frequencies of categories within texts which can be represented numerically and analysed by computer (Berelson, 1952). This method continues to enjoy popularity as a means of analysing the frequency of messages or particular depictions in media texts. It can provide a starting point for documenting the manifest or obvious messages in a group of media items, and for detecting patterns in a large mass of data which might otherwise not be obvious. However, while such analyses of textual content are useful for providing enumeration of obvious categories, they tend not to provide detailed accounts of the micro properties of the language used or identify the discursive formations and ideologies evident in news reports. Such analyses are largely limited to description, and are constrained in their ability to provide critical explanations of why medical and health issues are framed in certain ways and not others.

As shown in the previous chapter, the insights of critical analyses of AIDS as news have given greater depth to the generalizable findings of quantitative content analyses, providing a further socio-political and historical dimension to the understanding of AIDS as a cultural phenomenon. Such studies have emphasized the importance of the choice of language and topics in news accounts by which AIDS issues are framed and given meaning, demonstrating that AIDS is indeed an 'epidemic of signification' (Treichler, 1989), and that any attempt to understand the social construction of the disease must be cognizant of the properties of AIDS discourses in both the public and the private domains, how 'time and time again . . . the epidemic has been used to articulate values and beliefs that have nothing to do with AIDS' (Watney, 1989c: 19). This chapter outlines the method of analysis, critical discourse analysis, that was used to study the use of language in Australian newspaper accounts of AIDS. This method combines elements of systematic content analysis with a more interpretive and in-depth examination of the properties of news texts.

The structure of news

Health professionals and advocacy groups who criticize the news media's treatment of health and medical issues have tended to judge it according to their own agenda, that is, to disseminate accurate information about risk factors and encourage adherence to preventive health practices. However, such criticisms tend not to take into account the imperatives of journalism. Journalists, camera operators and producers report the news according to their own principles of newsworthiness, which involve rational strategies and decision making (Colby and Cook, 1991).

To understand the ways in which news is produced, it is important to consider the various constraints and demands upon newsmaking bodies. News in the capitalist world is often a commodity, used to sell advertizing: it is 'a depletable consumer product which must be made fresh daily' (Tuchman, 1978: 179) and which must make money in the process. This feature of news has an impact upon the selection and framing of events considered newsworthy, and in many cases acts as a limit to the scope of news. News must also entertain to sell newspapers, and to keep the audience's attention. It therefore must be compatible to the needs and interests of audiences. Furthermore, news-making bodies must also please their advertizers, who have the power to withdraw their financial support if they do not like the political stance of news reports (Philo, 1983: 132–3).

The economic pressures of the market dictate that there must be news every day. A single event is therefore more likely to be reported than a long process (Fowler, 1991: 14). In addition, this news must fit into the space allowed it; a certain number of minutes in a television news broadcast, or columns in a newspaper. Time constraints also mean that journalists often rely upon known sources, or 'experts' to give opinions quickly, rather than search for alternative views. In medical and health reporting, journalists must deal with constantly changing events and scientific evidence, and present complex information in a way that will be readily understood by the audience. There is little time for in-depth research into health issues, and therefore journalists tend to rely upon known sources of technical information, people or interested groups who are willing to give their opinion (Nelkin, 1987, 1991; Klaidman, 1990, 1991).

Several characteristics of 'good news' are influential in determining the shape of reporting of issues and events. Of all the myriad of events which happen in the world each day, only a minuscule number is selected as 'news'. As Hall, Critcher, Jefferson *et al.* (1982: 53) assert: '[t]he media do not simply and transparently report events which are "naturally" newsworthy in themselves. "News" is the end-product of a complex process which begins with a systematic sorting and selecting of events and topics according to a socially constructed set of categories'.

Meyer (1990: 52) has identified several features of news: timeliness (news must be 'new'), proximity (especially geographical nearness), consequence (events that change or threaten to change people's lives), human interest (evoking an emotional response or demonstrating a universal truth), conflict, prominence and unusualness. Tuchman (1978), Fishman (1980) and Galtung and Ruge (1981) have identified similar characteristics: newsworthy events usually concern elite persons or nations, are dramatic, are novel, are of geographical or cultural proximity, are unambiguous, are unexpected, are extreme, are relevant, can be personalized, have negative consequences, are part of an existing newsworthy theme, can be attributed to valued news sources, and contain facts. Bell (1991: 159–60) adds the often paradoxical and competing values of continuity (once something is in the news it tends to stay there), competition (newsmakers value the 'exclusive', the 'scoop' story), co-option (a story which is only tangential can be presented as part of a high-profile continuing story), composition (editors want a mixture of different sorts of news), predictability (whether the event is pre-scheduled and expected) and prefabrication (a ready-made report or press release of a story will be more likely to be used as it saves the journalists work).

In response to the unwritten laws of newsworthiness, journalists tend to emphasize the dramatic or tragic elements of a story, and tend to focus upon events which happen in close geographical or cultural proximity. Thus events occurring in Britain or the USA tend to be considered more newsworthy by the Australian press than those occurring in Indonesia, Africa or China; and the death of one white person is more newsworthy than those of several black people. As well, news values mean that persons who are considered elite are given greater voice than others – they are 'prominent news actors' (van Dijk, 1991: 40). The choice of 'talking heads' can therefore determine the way in which events are interpreted by audiences and readers of news accounts, setting the agenda for discussion of an issue and on occasion influencing government policy. The more famous the news source or actor, the more likely this is to happen. As Rogers, Dearing and Chang (1991: 41) have suggested, '[a] US president can move the media on any particular issue. All he [sic] has to do is give a talk about it'. By contrast, the views of members of the general public tend not to be sought, except to provide a 'personal' dimension upon a story, so that their status as newsworthy is accidental (Fowler, 1991: 22). News actors routinely include the following archetypes: a political figure, an official, a celebrity, a sportsperson, a professional or other public figure, a criminal or the accused, a human interest figure, and a participant (for example, a victim or witness) (Bell, 1991: 194).

Studies that have examined the use of news sources in medical and public health stories note that government officials, medical journals and 'celebrity' authorities tend to receive the greatest coverage in press coverage of medical or scientific controversies (Shepherd, 1981; Karpf, 1988; Nelkin, 1987; Greenberg and Wartenberg, 1991; Ryan, Dunwoody and Tankard, 1991; Klaidman, 1991). For political reasons, the individuals who act as the intermediaries between the lay public and information on health risks, often exaggerate the dangers in the quest for public support for research and policy measures. Medical spokespeople are valued as news actors, but their celebrity standing is rarely as great as that of famous movie stars or elite sportspeople. Dr Christiaan Barnard, the first surgeon to successfully perform a heart transplant, is one of the few doctors to have achieved global fame.

One major feature of news stories which is particularly relevant to the framing of health news in the media is the use of quantification. It is considered important to include figures in news accounts, to substantiate statements and act as hard 'facts', for 'figures undergird the objective, empirical claims of news' (Bell, 1991: 203). Figures also serve a rhetorical purpose, enhancing the news value of a story and adding drama. Roeh and Feldman (1984), in their analysis of the use of rhetoric in two Hebrew daily newspapers, found that the papers routinely used numbers with other rhetorical devices such as alliteration or parallelism. They suggested that in addition to acting as agents of a rhetorical objectivity, numbers in news stories were also used to appeal to the audience's emotions, especially in the tabloid press. The authors asserted that the use of numbers contributes to creating the impression that human destiny is determined by external rather than internal forces, notably accident and coincidence (Roeh and Feldman, 1984: 366).

News as a social construction

For cultural studies scholars, news media accounts are like other cultural products, in that they do not merely reflect societal norms, values and ideologies but also serve to constitute them, as part of a complex and constantly reflexive relationship. It is commonly accepted that the media have the power to set the agenda for public discussion of issues, to decide what is important and should receive attention. However, more crucially, as Philo (1983: 142) argues, the media tell people not only what to think but what to think *with*, by controlling the type and extent of information available about an issue of which the audience often has no direct experience. What is considered important to include as 'news' is meaningful in itself, because news stories do not 'tell it like it is', but rather, 'tell it like it means' (Bird and Dardenne, 1988: 71). While news is not fiction, it is not reality, but a selective and edited story about reality. However, the privileged status that news has in our culture means that the information it presents is generally accepted as real, in a way information transmitted in a fictional drama series, for example, is not.

Commentators interested in the cultural determinants of news and how it fits into wider societal patterns focus analyse the way in which an event is framed must be 'meaningful' to the audience. News is a highly structured and patterned system of discourse. Events must be placed in some sort of context, form parts of a narrative whole, when they are reported as news. Schudson (1989: 279) conceptualizes this process as story telling, and sees news as a form of literature. Hall, Critcher and Jefferson *et al.* (1982: 54) regard the enculturation of news as the process of 'making sense' of events which are unpredictable, dramatic and unusual. By placing an event in context, journalists bring events into an already extant realm of meanings, or 'cultural map'. News is presented as novel, but yet linked in many ways to other events and reference systems (Hall, Critcher, Jefferson *et al.*, 1982: 54–5). In that way, not only do the news media define what should be considered important, they also define how to make sense of these events.

For an understanding of the way in which news contributes to everyday understandings of reality, it is important to go beyond the structural constraints of news production to examine the subtextual meanings of news. When newsmakers construct a news story, when they decide how to 'frame' the issue, they make choices from a range of discourses in their attempt to give meaning to the story. When journalists, like all producers of texts, construct their story, they attempt to resolve contradictions, to convince the reader as to the plausibility of their argument. These attempts are not always immediately apparent to the reader, but can be revealed by close examination of the discursive structure of the news account.

From the cultural studies perspective, power relations and dominant ideologies are reproduced at all levels of news-making in modern western society. Cultural theorists do not crudely insist that popular culture serves only to preserve the interests of the ruling class against a powerless and brainwashed audience, but that the ideologies supporting the status quo are generally reproduced in the mass media because the powerful own the media and their opinions receive privileged attention in the media. They argue that the resistance of the powerless to these dominant ideologies is generally, but not always, overcome by the taken-for-granted and subtle presentation of ideologies and their persuasiveness that they represent the 'true reality'. The 'conspiracy' theory of authorship of texts is rejected for a view which sees multiple and contradictory discourses as competing for attention in texts, yet within defined boundaries (Parker, 1992; Astroff and Nyberg, 1992). The critical analysis of the cumulative effects of the reproduction of power in the mass media, the ways in which meaning is conveyed, the sign-systems used to draw associations between objects, people, events or concepts by the news media, provides a key to understanding how the accepted reality is constructed in the public domain. The process serves to identify the often contradictory discourses competing for meaning in news texts, and seeks to explain why it is that certain discourses are favoured over others. It is this perspective upon news as a social construction that has been adopted within the analysis of discourses on AIDS in the Australian press which follows.

Critical discourse analysis

Confusingly, the term 'discourse analysis' has been used to refer to a varied collection of approaches to textual, and even non-textual analyses. In critical discourse analysis, the method used to examine texts is similar to that of the micro concerns of literary criticism combined with a broader sociological political perspective. Critical discourse analysis centres its attention upon the choice of words, the figures of speech and the style as well as the subject matter of verbal communications, and the manner in which meaning is reproduced therein. The method spends more time examining linguistic processes than most other textual analysis techniques in the cultural analysis tradition.

The term 'discourse' used here refers to language pattern and structure at a number of levels: conversations or written communication between individuals, talk or written communication at a group level, and mass media communication, both audio and visual, embedded in historical, political and cultural settings. A discourse is a coherent way of describing and categorizing the social and physical worlds. Discourses gather around an object, person, social group or event of interest, providing a means of 'making sense' of that object, person, and so on (Parker, 1992). Discourses are powerful, and have political functions, because they 'define, describe and delimit what it is possible to say or not to say (and by extension – what is possible to do or not to do)' (Kress, 1985: 6). The criteria for distinguishing discourses, as outlined by Parker (1992: 6–20), include the following: a discourse is realized in texts; a discourse is about objects, events, concepts or actions, e.g. an object such as a condom, a disease such as AIDS or an action such as sexual intercourse; discourses address the audience in a particular way, 'making us listen as a certain type of person' (Parker, 1992: 9); discourses are structured to persuade – they benefit or support some individuals, groups or institutions and oppress or attack others; discourses therefore reproduce power relations; a discourse is not discrete but refers to other discourses, overlapping in a complex inter-relationship; a discourse is historically located; discourses are therefore dynamic and changing. Discourses may be contradictory as well as complementary; for example, discourses of both hope and fear on cancer might be said to exist.

Because discourses attempt to persuade audiences to accept a particular version of reality over another, they are ideological. Using the word 'ideology' here does not refer to the concept of a false consciousness. Rather, throughout this book, the term is used more neutrally as defining a system of abstract shared beliefs, images or concepts which give structure to everyday life and which assist individuals to make sense of their world. Ideologies contribute to and shape the formation of discourses: in fact, discourses can be considered the realization of ideologies, the constellation of practices and verbal products by which ideologies are expressed, produced and reproduced. By their very nature ideologies are usually implicit and taken-for-granted. One of the tasks of critical textual analysis therefore is to uncover latent ideologies and to question their taken-for-granted nature and political use. The questions which should be asked at the ideological level of analysis include: what ideas, values, notions, concepts and beliefs are present in the texts, and which are absent? Whose voices receive attention over others? Whose interests are served by the reproduction of these ideas, values, notions, concepts and beliefs in the texts? How might audiences' view of the world be influenced by the texts? What kinds of stereotypes are perpetuated in texts? What norms and values are privileged over others?

Discourses have a specific symbiotic relationship to practices; they produce the types of practices that are adopted, and the practices themselves reinforce and contribute to discourses. For example, the discourse on surgery which portrays surgeons as heroes and saviours of life and patients as saved from certain death by medical technology, both supports and reinforces societal attitudes on the funding of high technology research and equipment. This discourse, which may be identified in sources as diverse as medical journal articles, the mass media, and in conversations between doctors and patients or among the lay population, also shapes the expectations that patients have when they seek medical care for health problems, the advice and treatment offered the patient by the medical practitioner, the career progression of the surgeon and the nature of instruction in medical schools. The discourse conflicts, and competes, with discourses that portray good health as a preventive issue, focusing on lifestyle modification rather than medical intervention as the preferred solution to disease and illness.

Compared to many other interpretive methodologies used in health research, the analysis of discourse is novel in taking the post-structuralist perspective which privileges the role of language in shaping people's ideas of reality and the social world and reproducing social norms of expected behaviour. Unlike other interpretive analyses of verbal communication, discourse analysis is highly conscious of the power relations inherent in any discursive formation. A high degree of self consciousness or reflexivity is therefore required in carrying out discourse analysis, incorporating an awareness that all knowledge is socially produced, that one is producing a discourse by analysing other discourses, and that one is inevitably writing from a certain political position. An important aspect to consider is choice. A discursive process always involves choice in its construction, and the inclusion and absence of options is significant, going back to the social context. The choice of words made is vital to the meaning of a communication, demonstrating on which side the speaker/writer is placing himself or herself; for example, when referring to an embryo as a 'foetus' or a 'person' or when calling a group of people a 'mob' or a 'crowd'. Another example is when AIDS activists demand that people living with AIDS not be called 'victims', where they are explicitly foregrounding the need to use language to represent such individuals as active, vital participants in society rather than passive, disempowered patients living out a death sentence.

The examination of texts is central to discourse analysis and other forms of interpretive cultural research. The commonsense everyday understanding of a 'text' is that it is a written artefact, generally commercially produced, such as a book. However, in the context of discourse analysis, texts are any tangible forms of communication that may be rendered in written form: bus tickets, tee-shirt or bumper sticker slogans, hospital records, computer games, in-house memoranda, electronic mail messages, letters as well as government reports, books, newspapers and magazines. Texts are not analysed in isolation, but regarded as links in an historical and ideological chain, from which meaning is drawn and culture reproduced. This approach acknowledges the 'intertextuality' of texts, or that texts are sites where meaning is produced from the interaction of the texts with other cultural forms (Fairclough, 1992). The critical analysis of discourse thus involves not simply a focus upon the words or phrases forming sentences, but upon the particular network of other discourses that can be identified as contributing to the meaning of the words. Features of AIDS discourses in the news media are therefore significant; they represent important choices, subconscious or otherwise, from amongst the myriad ways of framing AIDS as a news issue.

Micro analysis of news language

It should be emphasized that, as with other interpretive qualitative methodologies, there is no one 'correct' way to 'do discourse analysis'. Rather, there is a theoretical and ideological setting in which discourse analyses take place, and the way in which they are undertaken depends upon the researcher, the data and the research question. In critical discourse analysis, unlike quantitative research, the sample size is not necessarily a very important factor in critical analysis, for the primary focus of the analysis is upon the structure, style and persuasive features of texts and how these features reflect the socio--cultural context, rather than the statistical representativeness of the chosen texts (Potter and Wetherell, 1987: 161). While quantification may be used, it is very much secondary to interpretive, inductive analyses that draw on theoretical, historical and political bases. Indeed, depending on the direction of the discourse analysis, quantitative content analysis may not be used at all.

The quantity of data collected depends on the purpose of the analysis. A few exemplary extracts from relevant texts can more economically support observations than the tedious and redundant repetition of similar examples. However, it is important to be clear about the research problem and objectives, and to give a clear description of the nature of the texts used and why they were chosen. In all discourse analyses, regardless of their complexity, the emphasis is upon looking for patterns in the texts, for both consistency and differences in the content and form of accounts, for shared features, and for the function and consequences of accounts (Potter and Wetherell, 1987: 161).

Newspaper and magazine articles are rich sources of language suitable for analysis: the average newspaper may contain 100 000 or more words of text and it is very easy to 'drown in data' (Bell, 1991: 3). Press clippings are simpler to analyse than electronic media artefacts, for the latter use sound and image as well as words for effect, all of which need to be taken into account in an analysis. Because news accounts are complex texts, it is possible to examine many of their features in detail, including their superstructures, subjects and topics, headlines, editorials, use of argument, quotations and sources, and lexical, syntactic and rhetorical style; see van Dijk (1991) for a work which examines all of these features of news texts. Here, it was decided to analyse first the major topics and surface themes of articles about AIDS to give a broad picture of which issues were considered most newsworthy by the press, and second to concentrate upon the expressive features and lexical style of headlines, editorials and main text, with particular emphasis upon the use of metaphor.

The use of the word 'topic' designates a single event, action, person or group of people. For example, an International Conference on AIDS may be the topic of several news stories, as may be the death of a well-known person from AIDS, or the development of a new drug to treat AIDS symptoms. Topics are important in setting the agenda for which issues, events or individuals are considered important, and are demonstrative of subjective definitions of what constitutes a topic. Topics summarize complex information, and rely upon structured reference systems to provide meaning. They constitute what newsmakers consider to be the most important information about a news event (van Dijk, 1991: 71–3). The selection of the topics that receive major press coverage is the result of complex networks of professional, social and cultural ideologies which serve to reproduce the interests and concerns of powerful social groups. In the absence of other sources of information the press' decision to favour certain topics over others when reporting issues may be influential in defining the situation for audiences, and therefore serves political functions. For example, if the topics which feature in news accounts of AIDS tend to be concerned with the plight of people with AIDS who are heterosexual rather than gay, such a choice of topic may suggest that the former are considered more worthy of society's interest and attention than the latter. As this example suggests, an important aspect of documenting major topics is noting absences as well as presences, for what is omitted is as meaningful as what is included.

It is, of course, the case that many, if not all, news accounts will have more than one topic, but limits must be placed upon the extent of detail in which texts should be analysed, especially if they number in the thousands. Particular attention should be paid to the headline and lead sentence of the item. When a large body of news texts is to be analysed, listing major topics chronologically by month can allow a preliminary overview of which topics received ongoing attention in the press over several months, and which therefore may have had a greater impact upon framing the issue as news. This can be a useful way of examining whether the interest of the press in certain issues changed over time; or in other words, which issues the press considered 'newsworthy' or important for public discussion, and whose opinions were valued as being 'expert'.

The world 'theme' is used here to refer to a wide grouping of individual topics, to show the broader patterns in AIDS reporting. Topical themes provide the macro context within which topics 'make sense'. One topic may contribute to more than one theme and many of these themes are inter-related. For example, the topics concerning the development of specific new drugs and vaccines to treat or prevent against HIV infection may be grouped together into a topical theme entitled 'medical research on AIDS'. Chapter Six uses the term 'theme' in a slightly different way, to refer to the latent themes in which topics and surface themes are embedded. When used this way, they are referred to as 'subtextual themes' to distinguish them from topical (or surface) themes.

A news text can be considered to be 'like an iceberg of information of which only the tip is actually expressed in words and sentences' (van Dijk, 1991: 181). The remainder of the iceberg is comprised of assumed systems of knowledge and beliefs about the world which journalists and audiences must share if meaning is to be created. Topical themes (that is, the 'tip of the iceberg') position topics in a fairly overt system of meaning, related to certain sequences of events, other current events and general, local or world knowledge. Subtextual themes are more abstract and rely to a greater degree upon implicit ideologies, narratives and discourses for their meaning. Thus, the topical theme used as an example above, 'medical research on AIDS', may incorporate subtextual themes drawing on the ideologies and discourses of medical dominance, hope, the valorization of science and military imagery.

It is not only the topic which reflects ideological systems, but the language with which the topic is framed. The 'style' of a text gives hints as to the type of audience addressed, the speaker's social role and status, and the function of the text (van Dijk, 1984: 133). The 'genre' (the type of media product) of the print news media itself makes demands upon style to which journalists must conform. Newspaper reports are generally written in a certain style that makes them instantly recognizable as newspaper reports, and not, for example, other forms of brief published writing such as short stories or poems. The headline, the leading sentences, the grammar, the choice of words and phrases, the tone are all formulaic to the newspaper style. Different newspapers also have recognizable styles; for example, the style of a 'quality' broadsheet is often discernible from that of a tabloid newspaper, especially in such features as headlines and editorials, using smaller print, a greater number of words, fewer and smaller photographs and less dramatic and colloquial language.

'Lexical style' refers to the choices and variations of words made by journalists (van Dijk, 1991: 209). The lexicon (or 'mental dictionary') is the basic resource from which choices of words are made from the range available (Fowler, 1991: 54). Given that there is a certain limited range of words available in the lexicon, the choice which is made is highly important to understanding the meaning of texts. For example, people living with AIDS may possibly be described using any one or a number of the following terms: 'deviants', 'victims', 'innocents', 'promiscuous', 'survivors', 'battlers', 'homosexuals' or 'drug addicts'. AIDS itself may be described as 'a plague', 'a disease', 'a punishment', 'a disaster' or 'an enemy'. Each choice of term attempts to influence the way in which readers construct their knowledges and attitudes about the phenomenon in question.

Within these constraints of the newspaper genre, the lexical style is revealing. It is important to be aware of the use of implications and presuppositions in news accounts – i.e. the inferring of pre-existing knowledge and beliefs which need not be stated (van Dijk, 1991: 181) – as well as vagueness, denial, blame, comparison and contrast, understatement and hyperbole, stereotype, attribution, terms of abuse and endearment and irrelevance – all persuasive rhetorical devices that can serve to define the situation and present the perspective and interests of one group over another (van Dijk, 1991; Fowler, 1991). Recurrent patterns in describing things, events, groups or people should be identified, for they represent formulae or stylistic 'templates' that delimit the lexicon available to represent issues, and can cause different matters to be perceived as instances of the same thing and new incidences to be categorized using pre-existing formats (Fowler, 1991: 171–8).

Headlines are the most conspicuous part of a newspaper report,

and their main function is to summarize the most important information in the report. The headline is often based upon the content
of the lead sentences, which are used by the journalist to provide a
'hook' to attract the reader's interest and convey the substance of the
news story. Except for very small regional newspapers with a handful
of staff, it is usually the sub-editor rather than the journalist who wrote
the news story who takes responsibility for writing the headline.
Headlines often use colourful and expressive tropes (figures of speech)
in order to fulfil the functions of concise summarizing and capturing
attention. For example, consider the complex information in this lead
sentence:

> It may seem far-fetched to compare the epidemic of acquired immune deficiency
> syndrome that is sweeping the world with the black death (a form of bubonic plague)
> that in the 1300s wiped out a quarter of Europe's population. However, there are
> similarities that should concern everybody.
>
> *Canberra Times*, 7 April 1987

The sub-editor reduced this to three eye-catching, dramatic words:

A MODERN PLAGUE

Readers tend to read headlines first and only then the rest of the news
item. Headlines therefore may bias the understanding process through
their subjective defining of the situation (van Dijk, 1991: 50–51).

Editorials are also interesting press items, for they represent the
'official' voice of the newspaper. Editorials often briefly sum up events,
and therefore serve to frame the situation, again directing the audience to a certain selected meaning in a more obvious way than most
other channels of reporting. Unlike news reports, which are presented
as objective and factual, editorials overtly offer an opinion, and issues
may be described in evaluative terms, often with a moral statement
summing up at the end. For example, one editorial published in a
major Sydney newspaper concerning the threat of AIDS to heterosexuals (*Daily Mirror*, 6 April 1987) made such evaluative statements
as:

> Too many of us still think of AIDS as a tragic threat to a small, promiscuous section
> of the community . . . Nothing, of course, could be further from the truth. We are all
> in danger.

At the end of the editorial, it was suggested that 'a new morality – a
new, responsible recognition of the dangers of casual sex, one-night
stands, or multiple sex partners' is required to prevent the spread of

AIDS. The editorial concluded with the statement, 'AIDS is no longer something that only happens to others'. It is clear that the style of these statements is overtly opinionated, seeking to convince the readership to accept the 'truth' of the editor's standpoint that everyone is at risk from HIV infection. The use of the terms 'promiscuous', 'a new morality', 'responsible', 'casual sex' and 'one-night stands' convey the editor's view that not only are non-monogamous sexual encounters irresponsible and morally unacceptable, they are now life-threatening. The positions taken in editorials, as van Dijk (1991: 134) argues, 'are not personal opinions, but manifestations of more complex, socially shared, and dominant ideological frameworks that embody institutional relationships and power'. Editorials therefore comprise an important resource for the critical analysis of news texts, and the analysis here uses editorials extensively as empirical documents.

When considering persuasion in news texts, it is important to examine from whose perspective the topic is discussed, whose opinions receive prominence and which news actors and news sources are drawn upon. The use of direct quotation is revealing, for direct quotes from news actors or sources serve the purposes of demonstrating an incontrovertible fact, distancing the journalist from the opinions expressed, enhancing the credibility of the report, interpreting the events reported, predicting future events and adding colour and drama (Bell, 1991: 207; van Dijk, 1991: 152). If used by prominent news actors or sources, direct quotes (which are usually opinions rather than 'facts') may become news in their own right (van Dijk, 1991: 152). An example is an article published in the Melbourne *Herald* (20 May 1987) concerning the Roman Catholic Church's views on safer sex education campaigns promoting safer sex and the use of condoms. The article was headlined

BISHOPS CONDEMN 'CONDOM CULTURE'

and excerpts from the official statement prepared by Catholic bishops were directly quoted, including the following:

> We reject any form of education which relies on a single-minded promotion of prophylactics and fails to present moral responsibility and chastity as the true and best remedy.

This article was generated by the release of a prepared statement, and by virtue of the newsworthy properties of conflict and the high social status of bishops from the Catholic Church attracted the desired coverage to the Church's alternative point of view.

The choice of news actors and news sources can determine the way in which events are interpreted. For example, the opinions of minority groups are rarely reported, and if they do receive attention they are often presented as partisan, whereas elite news actors or groups are presented as 'neutral' (van Dijk, 1991: 153–4). If government ministers release media statements concerning AIDS policy, then they are likely to receive coverage in the news media because of their position. It is far more difficult for a community-based AIDS support group to attract the news media's attention to its media releases, and even if it does, the group's status as a fringe organization will usually mean that its statements carry little weight compared with those of a high-ranking MP.

Metaphor, long regarded as simply a rhetorical device, has reached a new prominence in the latter half of this century, as philosophers, critical theorists and linguists have revived interest in the function served by this type of trope. As Lakoff and Johnson (1981) have shown, metaphor allows us not only to convey meaning verbally, but to conceptualize the world.

Metaphors are systematic, involving categories of related metaphors. They work by demanding, by the principle of association, that objects or concepts are joined by their similarities rather than their differences. The establishment of such associations relies upon shared knowledge and belief systems to establish meaning. Metaphor therefore does not operate at the level of the word, but at the level of discourse. Metaphorical activity tends to take place around sites of difference, to be used in struggles over power, whenever there is ideological contention (Kress, 1985: 71). For these reasons, the identification of metaphorical systems is important in a critical analysis of news texts.

The use of metaphor has been particularly important in 'making sense' of AIDS during its construction as a new disease in the public consciousness (Sontag, 1989; Treichler, 1989; J.W. Ross, 1989). According to Ross' study of AIDS in the American press during the early 1980s, AIDS was explained using six main metaphors: 'AIDS is a plague' 'AIDS is death' 'AIDS is punishment for sin' 'AIDS as crime' 'medicine as war', and 'AIDS as the other'. Ross believes that the great danger of metaphor though is that it easily becomes an analogue or model, so that, for example, AIDS is believed not only to be like a plague in some ways, but shares almost all the characteristics of plague. The metaphor 'AIDS is death' allows little hope for those who have AIDS, while those of 'AIDS is punishment for sin' and 'AIDS as the other' serve to stigmatize people living with AIDS. Ross' analysis provides a basis upon which to compare the use of metaphor in Australian press accounts of AIDS.

The role of audiences

Unlike methodologies that rely upon scientific method and statistical procedures to demonstrate the validity and reliability of findings (such as quantitative content analysis), the methods utilized in critical discourse analysis rely upon the interpretive skills of the researcher for their verification. The interpretation of texts and other forms of communication is a problem both for quantitative and qualitative analyses of content, for there is 'nothing that can be called *the* content or *the* meaning of a communication' (Andren, Ericsson, Ohlsson *et al.*, 1978: 16, emphasis in the original). Researchers of audience response have contributed to developments in understanding how different audiences read texts by showing that there can be multiple dominant textual readings according to different social and historical conditions; see, for example, the work of Morley (1992). They have shown that meaning is not static: it will change as time goes by, for texts are 'sites around which a constantly varying and always many faceted range of cultural and ideological transactions are conducted' (Bennett and Woollacott 1988: 8).

Analyses of the meanings of a text should therefore be made bearing in mind that there is a world outside the text that actively influences meaning. Audiences may be viewed as bringing to the text a number of pre-existing discourses that are often determined by their own location in the social structure, for example, their social class, occupation, age or gender. First-hand knowledge, interpersonal interaction, other media products, class experiences and internal processes of logic may be resources used by audiences to resist or negotiate textual meanings (Curran, 1990: 152). Texts are therefore polysemic, capable of multiple meaning. Hence, a newspaper editorial which refers to gay men with AIDS as receiving retribution for their sexuality may be accepted as valid and sensible by a reader with fundamentalist religious convictions and homophobic views, but may be rejected by a gay man or liberal heterosexual who believes that all people have the right to express their sexuality as they like. Other readers may disapprove of homosexuality, but believe that AIDS should be viewed not as a punishment, but as a disease. Still others may have acquired HIV themselves, or know someone who is HIV antibody positive, and resent and actively resist the implication that HIV infection is a punishment and death sentence.

It is possible, however, to draw a distinction between the 'preferred' or dominant meaning of a message (the meaning that is intended by the originator of the message), the 'negotiated' meanings which result when audiences interpret the message, and the 'oppositional' readings which occur when members of the audience reject the preferred meaning (Hall, 1980). Texts are produced and read in conditions that are structured to some extent by discourses and genres which construct reading positions for audiences (Kress, 1985: 37). They are produced from a pool of common discourses and meanings, and are read within that framework of possible meanings. The more prominent an issue, the more it receives media attention, the more it is removed from the everyday experiences of audiences, the more reiterated are its ideological themes, the more likely it is that media representations are accepted by audiences. An argument may therefore be made for the utility of uncovering the preferred meaning as a way of understanding the dominant discourses competing for attention at the site of the text. Texts can be analysed in terms of their 'mode of address', or how the 'implied reader' is constructed and the audience positioned (Connell and Mills, 1985: 39). The text itself can be regarded as a signifier, a product of cultural meanings and values determined both by the specifics of its production, by the position from which it is produced and the audience it hails (Connell and Mills, 1985: 39).

Chapter 3

The Early Years of AIDS Reporting

The first AIDS patient to come to medical attention in Australia was identified and treated in November 1982. He was an American who was treated for *Pneumocystis carinii* pneumonia and eventually returned to the USA (Penny, 1988). The first Australian with AIDS symptoms was diagnosed in Sydney in March 1983 (Reid, 1988: 107). As in most other developed countries, in Australia the news media were central in first alerting people to the existence of the disease, and in shaping knowledges of the 'meaning' of AIDS. The gay press was the first to bring AIDS to the attention of its audience. On 3 July 1981, a one-paragraph news brief appeared in the Sydney gay magazine *The Star*, headlined:

NEW PNEUMONIA LINKED TO GAY LIFESTYLE.

The item noted that:

> A type of new pneumonia has been found in five young men, two of whom died, and may be linked to 'some aspect of homosexual lifestyle', according to the US Public Health Service's Center for Disease Control. Between October 1980 and May 1981 the five, all active gay men, were treated for pneumonia caused by the *Pneumocystis carinii* parasite. The center reported in its *Morbidity and Mortality Weekly Report* (*MMWR*): The fact that these patients were all homosexual suggests an association between some aspect of homosexual lifestyle or disease acquired through sexual contact and *pneumocystis* pneumonia.
>
> Galbraith, 1992: 18

Throughout the second half of 1981, gay publications continued to publish items about the disease, including the link that had been made between the use of amyl nitrite as a recreational drug and *Kaposi's sarcoma* in young American gay men. The tenor of such reporting implied that the disease was confined to a handful of cases in the USA and was not highly relevant to gay men in Australia (Galbraith, 1992: 19). It was not until 18 months later, at the end of 1982, that the gay press began to demonstrate awareness that this new illness was growing in seriousness for Americans and might become a problem for Australians. By May 1983, partly in response to the first diagnosis of immune deficiency in an Australian man, gay publications were discussing the importance of the disease for the Australian gay community. Coverage of AIDS in the gay press grew from that point onwards, providing extensive reporting of symptoms, treatment, community activities and prevention guidelines (Galbraith, 1992: 20).

Mainstream press attention to AIDS in Australia was slow in beginning; see Appendix 1 for an overview of the press in Australia. The first reports about the new illness were published in the Australian editions of two international news magazines, headlined

DISEASES THAT PLAGUE GAYS

Newsweek, 21 December 1981

and

OPPORTUNISTIC DISEASES

Time, 21 December 1981[1].

On 2 January 1982 the first Australian newspaper report appeared in the city generally acknowledged as the Australian centre of the gay community, Sydney. The *Sydney Morning Herald* noted in its headline, a

FATAL HOMOSEXUAL DISEASE LINKED TO LACK OF IMMUNITY

reporting that three studies had been published in the *New England Journal of Medicine* concerning a mysterious new disease. There was no more mention of the disease in the Australian press until 25 April that year, when another Sydney newspaper, the *Daily Telegraph*, printed an article headlined:

FEAR FROM CANCER THAT KILLS GAYS

with the observation that Sydney, given its large gay community, could be next to be affected by the disease. Again there was a relative silence for another few months until July 1982, when six newspapers, including those published in cities other than Sydney, published accounts of the new illness, and also warning that 'Australia could be next'.

Until the beginning of 1983, only 18 articles mentioning AIDS had appeared in metropolitan Australian newspapers. It was not until 1985, over three years after its first mention (as GRID) in the Australian media, that the press began to devote any significant attention to covering AIDS. However, in the four-year period between December 1981 and December 1985, the number of articles about AIDS published in the Australian press rose steadily. As shown in Figure 3.1, there was a near exponential increase in numbers of articles on AIDS published between 1983 and 1985. The vast majority of articles were published in 1985, when 3563 articles dealing with AIDS appeared.

As Figure 3.1 demonstrates, there were, however, definite peaks and troughs in the attention given by the press to the new disease. In 1983 there was a peak in numbers of AIDS articles in May, June and July: this peak corresponds to the first case of AIDS reported in an Australian resident. The attention of the press diminished for over a year, until July and August 1984, just after the identification of a specific virus as the cause of AIDS in May of that same year. Articles about AIDS in those months were characterized by an obsession with the dangers posed by infected blood products held in blood banks. During the 'Gay Plague' period, which French (1986) places from December 1981, when the first article mentioning AIDS in Australia was published, to October 1984, the focus of the press was almost exclusively devoted to the new disease and its effects upon gay men, the first group in which symptoms were identified. Headlines such as:

FATAL HOMOSEXUAL DISEASE LINKED TO LACK OF IMMUNITY
Sydney Morning Herald, 2 January 1982

FEAR FROM CANCER THAT KILLS GAYS
Daily Telegraph, 25 April 1982

NEW ILLNESS STRIKES GAYS
Launceston Examiner, 13 July 1982

'GAY PLAGUE' EPIDEMIC SWEEPING US
Australian, 17 July 1982

AUSTRALIA COULD BE NEXT ON THE LIST FOR THE 'GAY PLAGUE'
Australian, 19 July 1982

THE GAY PLAGUE – THE BIZARRE EPIDEMIC – AVERAGE VICTIM THE PROFESSIONAL MAN
Sunday Telegraph, 12 September 1982

clearly gave the message that the disease was confined to gay men. By this time, gay men were being refused medical and dental treatment in Sydney because of fears of casual contagion (Ballard, 1989: 355), even though no cases of AIDS had yet been diagnosed in Australia. By 1983, headlines provided some indication that other groups (mainly

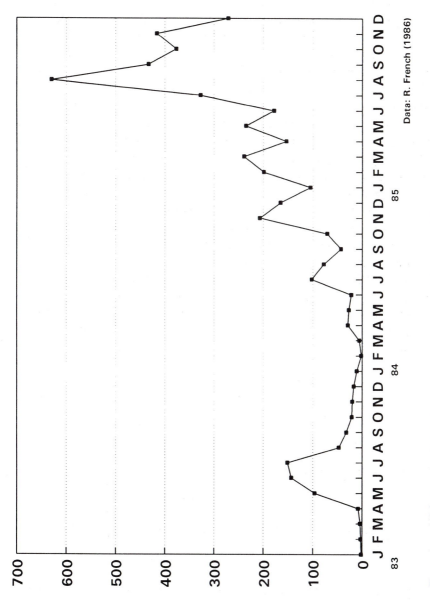

Figure 3.1 AIDS reporting in the Australian press, January 1983 to December 1985

those who had received infected blood products) might be at risk from the new and still mysterious disease:

HAEMOPHILIACS RISK DISEASE WITH ROUTINE TREATMENT
Australian, 15 February 1983

SEXUALLY TRANSMITTED BLOOD DISEASE MAY BE IMPORTED IN BLOOD TRANSFUSION PRODUCTS
Australian, 2 May 1983

DISEASE FEAR FOR CHILDREN
West Australian, 7 May 1983

AIDS PANIC HITS HEPATITIS VICTIMS
Sun, 26 September 1983.

However, the diagnosis of the first Australian (a gay man) with AIDS in April 1983 ensured continuing press focus upon the 'Gay Plague', and the following headlines appeared:

DISEASE FEAR LEADS RED CROSS TO BAN GAYS AS DONORS
Australian, 10 May 1983

SECOND CASE OF 'GAY PLAGUE' DISEASE DIAGNOSED
Australian, 11 May 1983

OPPOSING VIEWS ON TRANSFUSIONS – CALL TO HOMOSEXUALS TO NOT DONATE BLOOD
Canberra Times, 12 May 1983

W[estern] A[ustralia]'s HOMOSEXUALS WARNED ON AIDS
West Australian, 20 May 1983

FOURTH 'GAY PLAGUE' SUSPECT REPORTED
Australian, 26 May 1983

GAY COMMUNITY RESPONDS TO THREAT OF MYSTERY DISEASE
National Times, 26 May 1983

DOCTORS AND HOMOSEXUALS DISCUSS AIDS RESEARCH
Sydney Morning Herald, 27 May 1983

'GAY' KILLER GERM UNDER SURVEILLANCE
Illawarra Mercury, 5 June 1983

DISEASE 'STIGMA' FOR GAYS
Herald, 25 June 1983

AIDS DEATH HAS GAYS ON GUARD
Daily Telegraph, 11 July 1983

AIDS AND THE GAY DILEMMA
Australian, 25 August 1984.

The blood supply crisis

Although some official attention was given to AIDS after the first case of transmission of HIV by blood transfusion was confirmed in July 1984, the first major Australian government response was galvanized by the Queensland state government's announcement in November

1984 that three babies had died after receiving HIV-infected blood. Queensland subsequently passed legislation imposing criminal sanctions on people who failed to admit that they were in a 'high risk group' – at that time, gay or bisexual men with multiple partners, injecting drug users, and their partners (Ballard, 1989; 357) – when giving blood.

The focus of the press during this period was upon the death of the three Queensland babies infected by transfusions with HIV-infected blood, and on other 'innocent victims' infected by blood and blood products. Following the discovery of the infected infants in November 1984 there was another peak in reporting, and Bob Hawke, the then Prime Minister, was forced to appeal publicly for calm (Ballard, 1989: 357–8). Homophobic statements in the press were common, as gay men were accused of spreading HIV deliberately through donating blood. Headlines such as:

PLACE AIDS VICTIMS IN QUARANTINE: NILE

Advertiser, 15 November 1984

MOVES TO OUTLAW GAY BLOOD DONORS

Daily Mirror, 16 November 1984

GAYS ACCUSED OF BEING DONORS 'OUT OF SPITE'

Daily Telegraph, 17 November 1984

BLOOD ON THEIR HANDS

Daily Telegraph, 19 November 1984

SYDNEY'S HOMOSEXUALS IN FEAR OF REPRISALS

Advertiser, 20 November 1984

AIDS CARRIERS COULD BE CHARGED WITH MANSLAUGHTER

Hobart Mercury, 4 December 1984

MY BABY'S DEATH AGONY – AIDS DAD

Herald, 7 December 1984

'EXTERMINATE GAYS' – DOCTOR

Sunday Telegraph, 2 March 1985

introduced panic, fear and overt vilification towards gay men into AIDS discourse. One conservative politician was quoted in the *Australian* as saying, 'if it wasn't for the promotion of homosexuality as a norm by Labor, I am quite confident that the deaths of these three poor babies would not have occurred' (quoted by Ballard, 1989: 358) and Fred Nile, the leader of a revivalist religious group the Festival of Light, called publicly for the quarantine of all gay men (Ballard, 1992: 140). This era in AIDS reporting marked the beginning of the 'innocent' versus 'guilty' dichotomous categorizing of people with AIDS, with gay men and injecting drug users represented as 'guilty', and the recipients of infected blood products labelled 'innocent'. The *Sydney*

Morning Herald, one of Australia's most respected newspapers, published during this period an overtly homophobic account of the city's
annual Gay Mardi Gras. Other articles entertained the possibility that
swimming in pools which gay men had used, ear-piercing, tattooists
and mosquito bites could transmit AIDS.

In response to public outcry, an emergency meeting of state health
ministers was called. This meeting decided to reconstitute the existing
National Health and Medical Research Council (NHMRC) Working
Party on AIDS as the National AIDS Taskforce, led by Professor David
Penington, to provide scientific and medical advice to the Commonwealth government on the biomedical aspects of AIDS. Substantial
funds were pledged to the Red Cross Transfusion Service for screening
donated blood for HIV antibodies (Ballard, 1989: 358). The National
Advisory Committee on AIDS (NACAIDS), chaired by the nationally
well-known magazine publisher and editor Ita Buttrose, was also established in response to a decision made at the meeting (Reid, 1988:
106–107).

AIDS is personalized

Early in 1985 press attention returned to the 'Gay Plague' dimension
of AIDS, when controversy over the annual Gay Mardi Gras, held in
Sydney, was a major topic of articles. Press coverage of AIDS remained
reasonably high for the remainder of the year, as reports of the disease's
increasing incidence in Australia and other developed countries
continued to be published. In July, August, September and October
1985, the press' attention to AIDS leapt in terms of the number of
articles written about the disease. During these months the case of
Eve van Grafhorst, a small Australian child who was infected with HIV,
was a primary focus of the attention of the news media. Eve had
acquired HIV infection after receiving infected blood products. Her
infection became known in the small New South Wales town in which
her family lived, and moves were made to ban her from attending her
local kindergarten, for fear that she would pass on the virus by biting
other children. When Eve was allowed to return to kindergarten, several
children were withdrawn by their anxious parents. She was expelled
again after an accusation was made that she had bitten another child.
Eve's family was evicted from their house soon afterwards and experienced difficulties finding another house following objections by
neighbours. The van Grafhorst family eventually moved to New Zealand to escape the attention centred on the child. Headlines such as:

AIDS BABY – LITTLE EVE BANNED FROM A PLAY CENTRE
Daily Mirror, 19 July 1985

AIDS TOT SHUNNED BY KINDY MOTHERS
Daily Sun, 5 September 1985

CHILDREN BOYCOTT SCHOOL IN ROW OVER AIDS PUPIL
Australian, 11 September 1985

FORTY CHILDREN WITHDRAWN AS AIDS TODDLER RETURNS
Newcastle Herald, 30 September 1985

AIDS FEAR LEAVES EVE WITH A HANDFUL OF FRIENDS
Australian, 1 October 1985

THE TRAGEDY OF LITTLE EVE
Daily Telegraph, 26 October 1985

created a panic around the dangers of AIDS in schools, with other cases of infected children attending schools inspiring the following headlines:

AIDS PLEA: DON'T ISOLATE CHILDREN
Daily Telegraph, 20 July 1985

SCHOOLCHILD AIDS CARRIER
Hobart Mercury, 24 July 1985

AIDS IN SCHOOLS MAY STAY SECRET
Sydney Morning Herald, 27 July 1985

TEENAGER IS BANNED AT SCHOOL
Daily Mirror, 2 August 1985

AIDS CASE PANICS PARENTS OF CHILDREN AT SMALL UK SCHOOL
Australian, 2 September 1985

FEAR OF AIDS CAUSES HAVOC IN SCHOOLS
Australian, 14 September 1985.

Rock Hudson's illness and death from AIDS in October 1985, fears about AIDS in jails, the introduction of legislation in the state of New South Wales to impose penalties upon those who 'deliberately' spread HIV and the continuing 'Gay Plague' theme also resulted in a dramatic increase in AIDS articles during the closing months of 1985. The salacious details of Hudson's erstwhile secretive homosexual activities were revealed after the announcement in July that he had AIDS, and occasioned a multitude of headlines:

ROCK HUDSON'S TERMINAL CANCER LINKED TO AIDS
Australian, 25 July 1985

HOMOSEXUALS FIND A HERO IN HUDSON
West Australian, 27 July 1985

ROCK'S BOMBSHELL: THE NEWS THAT HE WAS GAY SMASHED AMERICA'S ILLUSION
Sun Herald, 28 July 1985

GIRL WITNESSED ROCK'S GAY 'WEDDING'
Daily Telegraph, 5 August 1985

HUDSON'S SECRET LIFE

Sun, 6 August 1985

HOW ROCK BECAME A HOMOSEXUAL

Daily Mirror, 9 August 1985

ROCK'S 'LOVER' SUES FOR $15M

Advertiser, 1 November 1985.

Throughout the early period of reporting, then, the focus upon gay men remained, with the occasional discussion of the problem of HIV infection via blood products. During 1985 there were a few headlines which suggested that heterosexuals could be at risk from AIDS through sexual contact:

AFRICAN STUDIES SHOW AIDS LIKELY TO INCREASE AMONG HETEROSEXUALS

Australian, 27 March 1985

AIDS SPREAD LINKED TO PROSTITUTES

Sydney Morning Herald, 4 May 1985

AIDS 'NOT A GAY DISEASE' IN AFRICA, RESEARCHER FINDS

Australian, 22 August 1985

MOST AIDS VICTIMS HETEROSEXUAL, WORLD CONFERENCE TOLD

Australian, 7 September 1985

HETEROSEXUALS AT RISK: STUDY

Launceston Examiner, 25 October 1985

MARRIED AIDS RISK

Sun, 10 December 1985.

However, there were less in number compared with those insisting that AIDS was a disease of gay men and blood-product recipients only.

AIDS and metaphor in the early years

The fundamental importance of metaphor in the context of AIDS is the establishment of novel connections, and hence, new meanings, to 'make sense' of the new disease. Sontag's (1989) essay focusing upon AIDS discourse commented upon the use of military, science-fiction, Biblical, invasion, assault, plague and punishment metaphors to give AIDS meaning. As she notes, 'AIDS has turned out, not surprisingly, to be one of the most meaning-laden of diseases' (Sontag, 1989: 179–80). Watney (1989c) has identified two major models of metaphorical thinking in health education approaches towards AIDS and news accounts of the disease. One is the 'Terrorist Model', in which HIV is conceptualized as 'an external invader, an illegal immigrant shinning up the white cliffs of Dover, a dangerous alien subversive slipping into the country unnoticed through Heathrow or JFK Airport, an enemy submarine sliding invisibly underwater under the belly of a fjord'

(Watney, 1989c: 20). According to Watney, this model condones the use of HIV antibody testing as a means of identifying the unseen invader before it has a chance to enter and destroy. The other metaphorical model identified by Watney is the 'Missionary Model'. Here, HIV infection is seen as a 'heathen entity, strange and exotic – thriving on immorality, bestiality, unnatural acts and ungodly practices, of which it is also seen as a product' (Watney, 1989c: 20). Watney argues that the solution to AIDS posed by adherents to this model of thinking about AIDS, is to return to Judaeo–Christian values and their attendant institutions – church, marriage, the family.

Scanning the early headlines of articles about AIDS reveals that, as was the case of the American press (J.W Ross, 1989), reports printed in Australian newspapers were characterized by at least eight main metaphors used to describe the nature of the first victims of the disease (gay men), the fatal nature of AIDS, and the fact that the cause of infection was unknown for several years. The metaphors most used in early AIDS reporting included: 'AIDS is gay', in tandem with 'AIDS is deviance' 'AIDS is a plague' 'AIDS is a mystery' and 'AIDS is death'. Other metaphors used as the epidemic progressed and worsened included: 'AIDS is an enemy' and the related metaphors 'AIDS is a violent attacker' and 'AIDS is a killer'. From the beginning of the epidemic then, AIDS was rhetorically framed in the Australian press as a lethal, violent, enigmatic, plague-like disease caused by homosexual 'deviance'. Common noun phrases used in headlines routinely employed such metaphors: 'fatal homosexual disease . . . homosexuals warned . . . gay plague suspect . . . gay killer germ . . . AIDS carriers charged . . . panic . . . disease fear'; a lexical formula into which subsequent coverage of the syndrome could slot.

Summary

Over the four-year period spanning the end of 1981 and the end of 1985, certain discourses and a defined AIDS lexicon developed in Australian news coverage similar in many respects to those extant in other western nations. The vilification of homosexuality, the drawing of distinctions between 'innocent' and 'guilty' people with AIDS, the panic over casual contagion, the interest in famous people who had developed AIDS, the denial of risk to the 'general population' and the metaphors associated with plague, death and divine retribution, were all evident in Australian press accounts of AIDS during this time. By 1985, the Australian press had contributed to the construction of a set of binary oppositions by which AIDS and its 'victims' could be identified:

AIDS/non-AIDS
homosexual/heterosexual
the other/self
punishment/reward
deviance/normality
guilt/innocence
male/female
death/life
bad blood/good blood
danger/safety
illness/health

However, in 1987, discourses on AIDS in the Australian press were to change dramatically, as the next chapter demonstrates.

Notes

1   All observations relating to press coverage in this section on AIDS reportage between 1981 and 1985, unless otherwise indicated, draws upon an annotated listing of all Australian newspaper and magazine articles on AIDS appearing between December 1981 and December 1985 published by Robert French (1986). This resource lists article headlines with publication and date details, and provides brief comments summing up their content. Given that only the headlines are available, the analysis in this section focuses upon these features only.

Chapter 4

The 'Grim Reaper' Period of AIDS Reporting

Despite the growth of warnings concerning the risk and incidence of HIV amongst all sectors of society in both the medical and the popular media, it was not until 1986 that the governments of developed countries began to consider heterosexual transmission of HIV as a real threat. During that year and into the next, reaction was strong on the part of health professional and government bodies in western countries to the increasingly highly publicized and documented threat which AIDS might pose to the 'general population', i.e. those people not classified as homosexual or injecting drug users. The prevailing sentiment in Britain was that the public had to be educated as a matter of urgency, before it was too late. Berridge and Strong (1991: 163) have likened this period in Britain to that of wartime emergency, when AIDS came to be seen as a 'potentially national crisis of epidemic proportions'.

In Australia, the risk of heterosexual transmission of HIV was placed firmly on the political agenda following a major AIDS Conference in Paris in June 1986, from which Professor David Penington, head of the National AIDS Taskforce, returned convinced of the need for a campaign to make the general Australian public aware of the risk posed to it by HIV infection (Ballard, 1992: 145). NACAIDS subsequently appointed a steering committee to survey needs and design an education programme. A benchmark survey was commissioned by NACAIDS to determine levels of knowledge about HIV and AIDS among Australians and was conducted in late 1986. The study found that 'although most people perceived AIDS as a threat to the nation, few saw it as a personal threat. The attitude that AIDS was somebody else's problem was highly prevalent' (Commonwealth Department of Community Services and Health, 1988). A national education campaign was therefore designed to create awareness of AIDS among all members of the Australian population. Funding in the order of approximately $3.63 million was provided. The primary aims of the campaign (and subsequent campaigns aimed at the general public) were:

> to provide clear, factual information to the public, in order to raise their (*sic*) general level of knowledge of AIDS and how it is transmitted; and to motivate the public to avoid practices that spread HIV infection (i.e. to avoid risk behaviours).
> Commonwealth Department of Community Services and Health, 1988

On 2 April 1987, the then Minister for Community Services and Health, Dr Neal Blewett, made a Ministerial statement to the House of Representatives in which he stated that 'it would be bordering on the irresponsible to ignore the objective facts and not undertake a full frank public education programme' (Crawford, Kippax and Tulloch, 1992: 7). Three days later, the controversial 'Grim Reaper' campaign was unveiled to the public.

Declaration of war: the 'Grim Reaper' campaign

The first Australian government-sponsored health education campaign aimed at the general public became known in popular parlance as the 'Grim Reaper' campaign because of the central icon employed in mass media advertizements. The imagery used in the campaign attempted to mobilize a fear and shock reaction similar to that aspired to by the British 'Don't Die of Ignorance' campaign run in 1986. This earlier British campaign had used the forbidding images of massive tombstones carved with the word 'AIDS', volcanoes and icebergs to convey the idea that AIDS was a hidden threat to everyone (Rhodes and Shaughnessy, 1990). Television, cinema and print advertizements for the 'Grim Reaper' campaign drew heavily upon medieval and horror movie imagery, portraying the grim reaper, a horrifyingly skeletal and skull-headed figure swathed in a black hood carrying a scythe and (incongruously) a bowling ball. Instead of ten-pins, a collection of stereotypes representing the diversity of 'ordinary' Australians were knocked down (killed) by the huge bowling ball aimed by the figure of Death. These included a housewife, a baby, a little girl, and a footballer. The intention was to render the abstract notions of death, danger and risk more familiar, and to demonstrate that people are like ten-pins before AIDS, vulnerable and powerless to protect themselves (Tulloch, 1989). Later scenes showed a band of grim reapers aiming bowling balls at similar groups of people to signify the potential of the threat to spread quickly. An ominous voice-over warned that all sexually active individuals should use condoms.

Print advertizements in newspapers and magazines supported the television campaign, reproducing a photograph of the main grim reaper figure. The print advertisements warned that:

> Anyone can get AIDS. It doesn't matter who you are, it's what you do that counts. At first it seemed that only gay men and IV drug users were being killed by AIDS. But now we know all sorts of people are being devastated by it. The fact is, experts say that in Australia over 50 000 men, women and children now carry the AIDS virus.

Accompanying press releases from NACAIDS emphasized the message, one of which (marked for release on 5 April 1987) included the following extreme statements designed to capture press attention and arouse the desired controversy:

> TWO MILLION AUSTRALIANS ARE NOW AT RISK FOR AIDS, SURVEY SHOWS — NATIONAL AIDS EDUCATION CAMPAIGN LAUNCHED TO WARN AUSTRALIANS THAT 'PREVENTION IS THE ONLY CURE WE'VE GOT' — SAFE SEX, SINGLE PARTNERS, ABSTINENCE, EDUCATION, CAUTION AND CONDOMS WILL PREVENT THE FURTHER SPREAD OF AIDS, SAYS ITA BUTTROSE.

> A major Government advertising campaign to inform and alert Australians about AIDS was launched today as a new survey of 'at risk' sexual and other behaviour showed that more than 2 million adult and adolescent Australians are candidates for exposure to the AIDS virus. The nation faces a major heterosexual epidemic of AIDS unless Australians radically change their sexual behaviour, says the Chairperson of NACAIDS, Miss Ita Buttrose . . .

The 'Grim Reaper' campaign received much publicity and media attention, especially during the week following the first showing of the television commercial. In the months leading up to the release of the campaign, the chairperson of NACAIDS, Ita Buttrose, herself a prominent journalist and editor and one of Australia's best known women, headed an effective pre-release publicity campaign that attracted press attention. When the 'Grim Reaper' advertizement was finally shown on 5 April 1987, the expectations of the waiting audience had been primed.

The release of the campaign marked the introduction of a new phase in media reporting of AIDS and of public anxieties about the disease. The commercial ran for only three weeks on television and six weeks in the print media but has become one of the most controversial and well-remembered advertizements ever shown, as was demonstrated by one study conducted three years after the screening of the campaign which found that the 'Grim Reaper' was the single most recalled message or story about AIDS amongst a randomly selected population of Sydney residents: 73 per cent in 1988 and 72 per cent of the respondents in 1989 still recalled the television advertizement (Bray and Chapman, 1991). During the running of the television commercial, some 40 000 telephone calls were received by the hotline established to deal with inquiries (Commonwealth Department of Community Services and Health, 1988). Heterosexuals flocked to clinics to have HIV antibody tests, the vast majority of whom were at little risk of contracting the virus (Mortlet, Guinan, Diefenthaler *et al.*, 1988).

The press response

The 'Grim Reaper' period of AIDS reporting was marked by an intensification and dramatization of AIDS coverage by the news media which is unlikely ever to be repeated[1]. The total number of press items referring to AIDS during this two-year period neared 9000 (8976). As shown in Figure 4.1, in terms of number of items published in the metropolitan Australian press, AIDS received an unprecedented amount of attention in the months (February and March 1987) leading up to and following the release of the campaign. The campaign generated much public controversy and debate. An enormous number of AIDS-related articles, features and letters to the editor were published in the print media in the weeks following the first showing of the commercial. For example, the number of articles printed in the first half of 1987 (3440) was over two and a half times that of the preceding six months (1341). In the month of April 1987 alone, 940 newspaper reports mentioned AIDS, the great majority of which were concerned exclusively with the campaign.

As Figure 4.1 shows, following this peak in AIDS coverage the number of articles decreased steadily until October 1987, although generally remaining higher than in pre-'Grim Reaper' months. Appendix 2 lists the major topics and number of news items by month appearing in the Australian press during this period of reporting. As the list of major topics demonstrates, the 'Gay Plague' theme continued to be evident in AIDS reporting in late 1986. The main topics considered newsworthy by the print media during this time were those to do with personalities ill or suspected to be ill with AIDS, infected by homosexual contact (Boy George, Freddie Mercury, Rock Hudson, Liberace, Prince Charles' valet), bizarre oddities (bedbugs may spread AIDS in Africa, person with AIDS is buried sealed in a concrete tomb), and scientific 'breakthroughs' on vaccines and treatment drugs. None

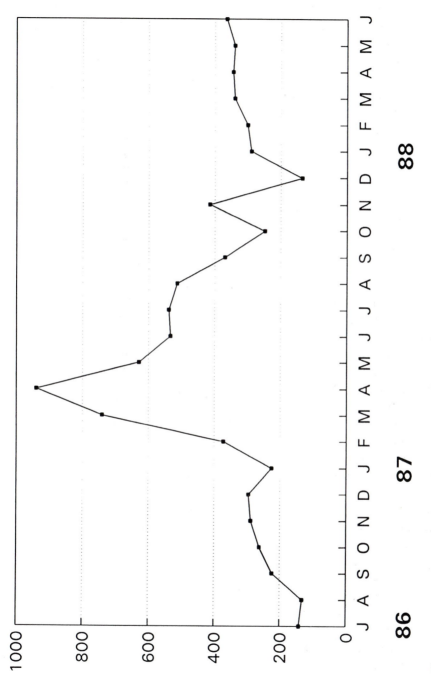

Figure 4.1   AIDS reporting in the Australian Press, July 1986 to June 1988.

of these topics differed substantially from the types of topics appearing in headlines in the early years. However, a growing interest in the issue of the threat to heterosexuals of HIV infection was becoming apparent by late 1986. With the advent of the controversial 'Grim Reaper' campaign, new topics linked to this threat began to dominate previous topics and themes.

During the several months following the release of the campaign the vast majority of newspaper articles were supportive of the government's decision to use fear-arousing tactics to create an impact. It is interesting to note the extent to which NACAIDS' publicity was taken up in newspapers accounts, including the uncritical adoption of the tone and phrases used by NACAIDS and their advertizing agency in planning a campaign which would strike fear into Australians. NACAIDS' intentions, as stated in their news releases and at the press conferences held for the occasion, were reproduced faithfully in the press, often with little change in wording:

SHOCK IS CAMPAIGN'S WEAPON

If the chilling, 60-second AIDS 'Grim Reaper' ad shocks every Australian, advertising whiz Quentin Munro will be a happy man. 'We're pulling no punches,' he said yesterday of the $2 million ad campaign . . .

Daily Telegraph, 7 April 1987

Other articles dwelt lovingly upon the controversial grotesque imagery used in the television advertisement:

A bowling alley of death, haunted by a decomposing grim reaper bowling over men, pregnant women, babies and crying children was featured on national television last night as part of a $3 million AIDS education campaign. The 60-second commercial featuring the grim reaper, a macabre and dramatic rotting corpse with scythe in one hand and bowling ball in the other, is spearheading efforts by the National Advisory Committee on AIDS to educate Australians about the incurable disease.

Financial Review, 6 April 1987

Headlines positioned the government actively as the opponent of the AIDS enemy and centred on the 'hard-hitting' and 'warning' nature of the campaign:

AIDS WAR STARTS: 2 MILLION AT RISK

Age, 6 April 1987

COUNTERING THE AIDS SCOURGE

Newcastle Herald, 15 April 1987

SHOCK TACTIC TO AVERT AIDS CRISIS

Advertiser, 6 April 1987

SHOCK IS CAMPAIGN'S WEAPON

Daily Telegraph, 7 April 1987

AIDS CAMPAIGN WILL SHAKE AUSSIES' APATHY

Daily Telegraph, 22 January 1987

AIDS AD 'HARD-HITTING': GRIM REAPER'S WARNING

Sun, 6 April 1987.

Editorials in most major newspapers in the week following the release of the 'Grim Reaper' advertizement dealt with the subject. The sentiments expressed were, for the most part, also largely supportive of the campaign, despite (or because of) its shock tactics. Hence the *Newcastle Herald*'s editorial opined that 'It was reasonable for the opening government advertisement to emphasize fear, for AIDS is a swift and brutal killer' (15 April 1987). The editor of the *Adelaide News* approvingly commented that 'The provisional verdict must be full marks ... AIDS threatens to be a pandemic which, unchecked, could be as devastating as the Black Death ... The depiction of AIDS as the Grim Reaper is shocking – but all too accurate a portrayal of what today stalks Australia' (6 April 1987). An editorial in the *West Australian* (7 April, 1987) began with the words, 'Grim it is, but grim it has to be', going on to say that 'the severity of AIDS calls for the straightest of straight talking – and even a dose of shock therapy – to raise public awareness of the virus'. The Brisbane *Daily Sun* (7 April 1987) commented that 'The fact that the advertisement lived up to the warning from Federal Health Minister Dr Blewett that it was harsh and shocking, should be regarded as positive, not negative. We are dealing with a monster'.

The tropes used in headlines and editorials are revealing. The *Australian* and *Daily Telegraph*'s editorial headlines displayed a slippage between the AIDS campaign and AIDS itself, implying that the spread of the disease was serving some purpose:

AIDS: A NEEDED SHOCK

Australian, 7 April 1987

AIDS: SHOCKS ESSENTIAL TO SAVE LIVES

Daily Telegraph, 3 April 1987.

Editorials went on to call the campaign 'a necessary shock' and 'gruesome', with 'no holds barred' but one which should be supported by 'all caring people'. Other editorials referred to 'public enemy No 1', the 'launching' of the campaign to 'combat' AIDS, and the need for 'hitting home with the hard facts' (*Launceston Examiner*, 6 April 1987). The *Advertiser*'s editorial headline declared 'PLAIN SPEAKING NECESSARY (2 April 1987) and argued that 'In the war against AIDS plain speaking is our chief weapon. Information is our defence against a disease that as yet has no cure … Survival is the issue, and in this war, plain speaking must not become a casualty'.

This privileging of education as the primary 'weapon' against AIDS, and of the dissemination of 'hard' facts as protecting against harm, was evident in other editorials; for example:

> The national AIDS education campaign, to be launched on Sunday, is essential if the lives of countless thousands are to be protected … In the absence of a vaccine, prevention is the only defence. And people will learn how to stop AIDS only if they are told honestly, explicitly, even starkly … Some people may find the commercials shocking. That, too, is unavoidable …
>
> *Daily Telegraph*, 3 April 1987

Thus the majority of editorials reacted favourably to the NACAIDS campaign, praising the shock tactics used. Rhetoric which portrayed the campaign as a brave onslaught against a monstrous virus seeking to overtake the country was extensively employed. The editorials for the most part reflected, in an uncritical manner, both the intentions and extreme statements of risk used by government spokespeople. The editor of the *Financial Review* was one of the few to sound a note of caution, asserting that NACAIDS 'is walking a tightrope between the urgent need to improve public knowledge of the basic facts about the disease on one hand and the danger of over-killing with its scare-them-silly, horrific commercials, on the other' (8 April 1987). This editorial called into question the role of the state in trying to change the behaviour of its citizens, and questioned whether the scare tactics would prove effective. It ended with the words, 'One can only hope that the future AIDS campaign material will be less dramatic, more rational and more informative than that which is inundating our TV screens at present'. The *Courier-Mail* editorial (6 April 1987) made the same point: 'We should not expect too much from scare tactics. Otherwise the hotels would be empty, the tobacconists would be bankrupt, the airlines would be grounded and cars would be driven at a sedate 40 kilometres an hour and only in perfect visibility'.

The language used in press accounts of the 'Grim Reaper' utilized several main metaphors. The dominant metaphor the campaign was attempting to convey by the use of the 'Grim Reaper' icon was that 'AIDS is death'. The 'Grim Reaper' is a centuries-old icon of death, and thus the metaphor 'The Grim Reaper is death' became the dominant imagery of the advertisement, creating a new metaphor, that of 'The Grim Reaper is AIDS'. A still from the advertisement depicting the figure of the 'Grim Reaper' became illustrative of any issue to do with AIDS, even though NACAIDS or the campaign itself may not have been mentioned in the article. The grotesque and medieval figure of the 'Grim Reaper' thus became the definitive sign of AIDS, bringing with it its older meanings of death, famine and plague, and divine retribution.

The adoption by the press of the horror-movie genre used in the actual advertisements when describing both AIDS itself and the campaign was a noticeable feature of coverage during this period. The disease was presented in horror-movie imagery, using the metaphor 'AIDS is a monster'. Adjectives and noun phrases referring to the image included 'we are dealing with a monster ... AIDS is exposed in all its ugliness ... we face the AIDS spectre ... a shock ... chilling ... visually frightening ... gruesome ... the AIDS scourge ... a bowling alley of death, haunted by a decomposing grim reaper ... a macabre and rotting corpse ... the deathly visage that sprang from our television sets'. Another metaphorical way in which newspaper articles and editorials represented the threat of HIV or AIDS was to personify the virus and the syndrome. Thus the metaphor 'AIDS is a vengeful killer' featured commonly in articles: 'it can strike anyone ... the deadly virus ... AIDS is lethal ... strikes 12 more victims ... is a swift and brutal killer ... has gained its deadly foothold in Australia ... might hit children ... can attack women ... terrorizes the US ... strikes again ... has killed a third of its victims'. In response to this personification of the disease, tropes and adjectives used to describe the government's strategy against AIDS tended towards physical, sporting, violent, fist-fight imagery: 'countering ... hard-hitting ... shake ... jolt ... pulling no punches ... tactic ... no holds barred ... hit home'. The emphasis in press accounts was typically upon the shock value, violent and 'no-nonsense' approach of the advertisements, as conveyed by the above words and phrases and other dramatic descriptive words such as 'shock ... stronger line ... explicit ... chilling'. By the use of this language AIDS was positioned as a deadly crisis against which the state must aggressively marshall its defences.

Metaphors of war are very commonly used in medical and scientific discourse, and have been utilized often in the western press since the beginning of the epidemic in its descriptions of AIDS. One major war metaphor which has been current since the beginning of AIDS reporting and continued in prominence into 1987 and 1988 is that of 'AIDS is an enemy': 'we are all in a danger zone ... an AIDS crusade ... AIDS has the potential to kill more Australians than World War II'. In this conceptualization the 'Grim Reaper' campaign represented a fight or battle against AIDS, in which violent means were necessary to win. Commonly used words in press accounts were 'weapon ... kill

. . . strike . . . public enemy No 1 . . . aimed . . . combat . . . defence . . . survival . . . casualty . . . war'; even the word 'campaign' has military associations. The new metaphor 'Health education as weapon' to combat the 'AIDS enemy' thus appeared in the press, challenging more traditional metaphorical representations of medical science as the primary protagonist in waging war against illness: 'Prevention is the only defence . . . plain speaking is our only weapon . . . our only weapon at the moment is education . . . knowledge answer to killer AIDS . . . information is the only weapon we have against AIDS'. It is significant that this metaphor gained prominence in the months leading up to and following the 'Grim Reaper' campaign. Until that time, AIDS education directed at gay men was given little press attention, and no other mass media campaigns directed at AIDS education and awareness existed.

Such rhetoric not only served to position AIDS as the enemy, against which both the tactics of one-to-one combat and full-scale military war should be used, but also to position the government in a paternal, dominant role. Health education was largely depicted as a 'top-down', 'one-way' exercise with those at the top (government authorities) attempting to disseminate the knowledge about risk to those at the bottom, the ignorant members of the public who could not be trusted to disport themselves wisely because of their lack of knowledge. According to this rhetoric, the Australian public was also positioned as 'the enemy' because of its complacency, apathy and ignorance. The state was unambiguously placed in the traditional model of authority figure wielding discipline over the unruly, taking a 'stronger line' and threatening the punishment of death if the message were ignored: 'people will learn how to stop AIDS only if they are told honestly, explicitly, even starkly'. The role of the state was little questioned in press accounts. Debate concerning the public's rights to control over its own sexual conduct, the accuracy of the statistics and epidemiological predictions upon which the warnings were based, or the government's right to incur anxiety, fear and guilt in the Australian population using shock tactics to 'destroy complacency' were absent in the vast majority of reports.

The discourse of AIDS risk during this period therefore privileged a 'knowledge' of HIV transmission and an 'awareness' of personal risk. These concepts were unanimously portrayed as positive, for they constituted the only 'weapon' against the spread of AIDS. This stance effectively devolved responsibility from the state for the control of AIDS to the individual; the state was seen to do its job in publicizing the danger and threat associated with AIDS in the strongest possible terms and then leaving it to individuals to respond in the manner deemed appropriate.

Ita Buttrose, radical celibate and new 'AIDS expert'

An important and dominant feature of AIDS reporting during the 'Grim Reaper' period was the use of direct quotes from a select coterie of 'AIDS experts' to support or provide dramatic statements and headlines. The opinions of Ita Buttrose, the Chair of NACAIDS, were quoted extensively with reference to the threat to heterosexuals of AIDS. Buttrose's personal community standing, her many years in journalism, her access to the press, all combined to ensure that the message of the 'Grim Reaper' campaign would be highly publicized and supported by the popular press. Although having no previous direct connection with AIDS issues, and despite the fact that she had no medical or research training at all, by virtue of her community standing as an established and respected 'personality' Buttrose was able to engender enormous publicity for the cause, and her name and photograph were widely published in articles about the threat posed by AIDS to the Australian population.

As the headlines below demonstrate, many of Buttrose's pronouncements concerning the risk to heterosexuals of AIDS were faithfully reproduced as if she were a quasi-religious leader offering a miracle solution to the epidemic. Headlines often referred to Buttrose by her first name only, presupposing her renown, and at the same time, personalizing her and implying a degree of familiarity. They also portrayed Buttrose as a dynamic leader, with expert knowledge and judgement which should be followed:

AIDS KNOWS NO BOUNDS: BUTTROSE

Hobart Mercury, 19 June 1987

ITA THE FIGHTER: ONE WOMAN'S WAR AGAINST PUBLIC ENEMY NUMBER ONE

Daily Mirror, 6 April 1987

AIDS A THREAT TO ALL: ITA

Sun, 8 December 1986

IT'S ITA'S AIDS REMEDY: SAY NO

Sydney Morning Herald, 6 April 1987.

Buttrose was routinely portrayed in the press as a tireless worker against the dangerous enemy, and as an authoritative, almost bossy leader in the 'school-ma'am' or 'strict mother' model. Her statements about the risk faced by all Australians tended towards the conservative, the moralistic and the dictatorial, and her pronouncements were often used as direct quotes, for example:

> Too many Australians believe they will not be affected by AIDS, according to Ita Buttrose . . . Miss Buttrose said she was 'astounded' at the attitudes that many Australians have towards the disease. 'While 98 per cent of Australians say there should be an education campaign, far too many believe that AIDS won't affect them – they feel that it is everyone else who is at risk of the disease,' Miss Buttrose said. 'This is a very selfish attitude, as it is proven that everyone is at risk from AIDS.
>
> *Sun*, 8 December 1986

> [Buttrose said] 'Abstinence is the best way to stop the spread of AIDS. Fidelity in marriage is vital – so are one-to-one relationships. The message that must be absorbed is: if you don't know where your partner has slept before he or she sleeps with you, then don't. If temptation is too hard to resist, then use a condom'.
>
> *Sydney Morning Herald*, 6 April 1987.

> AIDS campaigner Ita Buttrose yesterday laid down the new golden rules of sex. Casual sex and one-night stands were out and multiple sexual partnerships downright dangerous, she said at the launch of a new AIDS education campaign.
>
> *Sun*, 6 April 1987

In these excerpts, the statements attributed to Buttrose are didactic and imperative, giving a clear, pared-down and simplistic message of 'correct' behaviour that resonates with former First Lady Nancy Reagan's motto of 'Just say "No"' in response to illicit drug use. In these accounts Buttrose is portrayed as lecturing the public in matters of personal hygiene. Members of the public are once again positioned as 'naughty schoolchildren', needing discipline and firm guidance to protect themselves from their 'selfish attitudes' and their inability to resist temptation.

One example is a media text in which Buttrose used her regular column (entitled 'Ita's Page') in a popular women's magazine to proselytize. The ideologies of paternalism and utilitarianism are dominant in the article, which is headlined

DEFEATING AIDS IS EVERYONE'S RESPONSIBILITY

Woman's Day, 2 March 1987.

Buttrose spends the bulk of the article drawing comparisons between Africa and Australia. After describing the extent of the AIDS epidemic in Africa, and emphasizing that HIV is spread there 'mainly through heterosexual transmission', Buttrose draws further parallels between the extent of unemployment in Africa and Australia, the AIDS issues addressed by governments in Africa compared with those addressed by NACAIDS, the role of churches in both continents in 'fighting the spread of AIDS', and the desire of both to 'determine their own policies and approaches to AIDS'. The clear implication is that Australia faces similar devastation from AIDS to that currently experienced in parts of Africa if strong measures are not taken.

Buttrose emphasizes the responsibility Australia has to help developing nations deal with the threat of AIDS. She then moves abruptly to the attitudes of Australian men to AIDS, implying that just as Australians need to help other countries, so too they need to address the problem of AIDS in their own country, and 'take the necessary precautions'. The article ends by placing the responsibility upon women all over the world to ensure safer sex practices are followed: 'women will have a vital contribution to make, not just in Australia, but also the rest of the world, in persuading their partners to use condoms'. Buttrose pre-empts any criticisms that women should not have to take responsibility for saving the world from AIDS by noting; 'Some feminists may grumble that women shouldn't have to take responsibility for safe sex, that men and women are equally responsible. Unfortunately, AIDS is too serious a threat to become caught up in arguments about equality'. The headline and the final phrase of her Churchillian advice in this column emphasize Buttrose's public single-mindedness in her role as the disseminator of the 'right' message: 'Stopping the spread of AIDS supersedes all other considerations – and we all have a role to play'.

Buttrose's announcement during this time that she was a 'radical celibate' added both authenticity and controversy (and hence, newsworthiness) to her assertions that 'casual sex is out' and 'fidelity in marriage is vital', and bolstered her portrayal as a conservative matriarch or spinster school teacher figure. Several headlines capitalized on this:

WHY ITA SAYS NO TO SEX – FOR NOW

Sun, 9 April 1987

FREE LOVE IS OUT, SAYS CELIBATE ITA

Advertiser, 6 April 1987

ITA: WHY CELIBACY MAKES SENSE

Sun Herald, 5 April 1987

CELIBATE ITA LAYS DOWN SEX RULES

Sun, 6 April 1987.

Buttrose was thus able to offer her own sexual behaviour as a shining example to others. Her self-proclaimed celibacy intensified her portrayal in news accounts as a quasi-religious leader, as did the moralistic tone of her preaching concerning the resisting of temptation, free love and selfishness, compared with the benefits of disciplined self-restraint, celibacy, abstinence, monogamy and fidelity.

Apocalyptic visions

In the 'Grim Reaper' period of AIDS reporting, apocalyptic warnings of how the virus would destroy civilization as we know it became common in press accounts and the metaphor 'AIDS is an apocalyptic disaster' entered into circulation. More specifically, now that it was being suggested that everyone was at risk from the disease, the metaphor 'AIDS is a latter-day plague' was often used. Unlike previous representations, the addendum 'gay' was not added to the phrase, suggesting again that all members of society were at potential risk of mass devastation by the virus. AIDS was no longer simply a disease of the 'other', but a disease which threatened to decimate the population. This change is an important one, which deserves detailed attention to the rhetorical devices used to convey this message in the press.

With the message that AIDS is waiting to destroy the world, came the metaphor 'sex is dangerous'. Unlike previous metaphorical representations of AIDS which espoused the danger of gay male sexual activity only, this metaphor implied that all 'promiscuous' sex, whether homosexual or heterosexual, was risky. During this period of AIDS reporting, the dominant metaphor 'AIDS is gay' therefore changed to 'AIDS is heterosexual'. The following headlines demonstrate the outcome of such a transition:

AIDS – THE PLAGUE OF THE 80S AND IT'S HERE TO STAY
Cairns Post, November 3 1986
AIDS: A TIME BOMB JUST WAITING TO BLOW LIVES TO BITS
Hobart Mercury, 10 April 1987
AIDS: HORROR TOLL'S SOARING, AND IT'S THE NEW BLACK DEATH FOR THE 21st CENTURY
Sunday Times, 8 February 1987
AIDS: KILLER PLAGUE
Daily Sun, 2 March 1987
AIDS IS A POTENTIAL HOLOCAUST
Sunday Mail, 22 March 1987.

Other headlines asserted that all Australians were at risk from HIV infection, and that the disease was spreading unchecked amongst all sections of the population:

AIDS SPECTRE NOW BECOMES UNIVERSAL

Age, 21 February 1987

AIDS: WE ARE ALL IN DANGER

Daily Mirror, 6 April 1987

AIDS OUT OF CONTROL HERE SAYS EXPERT

Daily News, March 2 1987

KILLER DISEASE CASTS DEADLY SHADOW OVER WORLD: AND ALL OF US ARE AT RISK

News, 17 February 1987

SYDNEY'S SHAME: AIDS IS SPREADING FASTER THAN FEARED

Sun Herald, 1 February 1987

AIDS ATTACK: RISK SPREADS TO 'STRAIGHT' PEOPLE

West Australian, 21 March 1987

'IT'S A THREAT TO EVERYONE – FROM BABIES TO SOLID MARRIED COUPLES'

Daily Telegraph, 5 April 1987.

Like the headlines current at this time, editorials and the main body of articles were almost universally pessimistic about the spread of AIDS, forecasting doom for all Australians, and emphasizing the fact that everyone was now at risk. The *News* (17 February 1987), for example, stated that 'Swingers of all sexual preferences are now at risk. Thus, as AIDS spreads rapidly through the heterosexual community, all of us are at risk, no matter our age, our sex, or our degree of loyalty to our sexual partners'; while the *West Australian* (21 March 1987) drew comparisons between the USA, Africa and Australia to incite anxiety in heterosexuals: 'AIDS will soon be a worry for young 'straight' men and women in Australia unless they change their ways. Doctors, noting the American and African experience, predict horrifying trends for sexually active heterosexuals'; and the *Daily Telegraph* (5 April 1987) warned that; 'the deadly AIDS virus has the potential to affect us all, not only homosexuals and drug users . . . AIDS is a threat to everyone from tiny babies to solid married couples . . . AIDS is spreading at an accelerating rate into the heterosexual community and worldwide more than half of all AIDS victims are heterosexual'.

Prevailing discourses on AIDS had changed markedly since the early years of reporting, from a discourse of risk centring around the specific and contained threat to reviled deviant outgroups, to a discourse which extended the risk wholesale to every individual, regardless of their sexual proclivities. Phrases and adjectives now depicted AIDS as a disease which was 'the AIDS crisis . . . out of control . . . the new black death . . . the plague of the 80s . . . here to stay . . . universal . . . tragic . . . a threat to everyone . . . one of the gravest threats to the health of Australians ever confronted . . . spreading at an accelerated rate into the heterosexual community . . . spreading faster than feared'. News accounts predicted that 'AIDS could wipe out the human race . . . a potential holocaust' and asserted 'we are fighting for survival against AIDS . . . we are all in danger . . . killer disease casts deadly shadow over the world'. There was little critical discussion in these panic-stricken accounts of the probabilities of contracting HIV infection. Rather, articles tended to state baldly that 'all of us are at risk', and 'death is a possibility for each and every one of us'. The emphasis in press reports was upon individual behaviour change, again supporting the primary message of NACAIDS and the Commonwealth Department of Community Services and Health that all individuals were responsible for stopping the spread of HIV in the Australian community. Statements of impending doom were thus coupled with the solution: individual behaviour change, as in the following phrases: 'very promiscuous people will all get the virus in the next five years unless they take precautions . . . unless they change their ways . . . prevent or protect themselves against exposure . . . defeating AIDS is everyone's responsibility'.

Again, typical imagery from the cinematic and pulp novel genres of horror, science fiction, suspense and thrillers were common, seeking to frighten and perhaps to titillate the audience. Part of the danger posed by the virus, according to the metaphor 'AIDS is a hidden danger', was that it moved in insidious ways: 'the AIDS scare is quietly simmering . . . the tip of the iceberg . . . an insidious enemy that lurks within . . . AIDS is quietly rampaging . . . an AIDS timebomb'. The use of such hyperbolic phrases, stereotypical and hackneyed as they are, suggests that the danger was being overstated for effect (and newspaper sales). The strong parallels with the genres of popular horror and suspense in this discourse has the effect of diminishing while simultaneously exaggerating the threat of the disease.

The use of quantification by 'AIDS experts' was a major element of the apocalyptic imagery dominating press accounts of AIDS during the 'Grim Reaper' period. Direct quotes from prominent news sources and news actors were a favoured means of presenting quantification rhetoric. Although Ita Buttrose received the most press publicity about her views on AIDS, high-profile Australian physicians, politicians and statesmen also served as news sources giving public warnings about the threat posed by HIV to the Australian public. For example, in late 1987 the Governor-General of Australia became an unlikely yet influential spokesperson for the cause, attracting headlines for his statements that AIDS would affect everyone:

CASES WILL INCREASE AT 'HORRIFYING RATE'

Governor-General Sir Ninian Stephen yesterday predicted the spread of AIDS would continue at 'a horrifying rate' . . . 'As this fatal infection spreads many of us will have friends and relatives who die of it,' he said.

Daily Telegraph, 22 July 1987

As the above excerpts demonstrate, the hyperbolic use of predicted numbers or proportions of HIV-infected people was a feature of many accounts and headlines which quoted the views of the 'AIDS experts'. For example, statements from the Australian Commonwealth Minister for Health, Dr Neal Blewett, were reported in the press warning that 'up to 50 000 Australians, most of them walking around in apparently good health, were in fact carriers of one of the most lethal viruses ever known' (*Sydney Morning Herald*, 2 April 1987). The opinions of prominent physicians also received press attention:

. . . there have been Sydney-based predictions of 50 000 people Australia-wide exposed to the virus who could be passing it on through sex or through sharing needles to inject drugs. 'Very promiscuous people will all get the virus in the next five years unless they take precautions,' says Dr Watson.

West Australian, 21 March 1987

Headlines predicting the fast spread of AIDS included:

AIDS: 2 MILLION AUSTRALIANS AT RISK

Australian, 6 April 1987

FEMALE HETEROSEXUAL CASES DOUBLE

Launceston Examiner, 18 April 1987

AIDS NOW AFFECTS 17 500 AUSTRALIANS: PENINGTON

Australian, 14 May 1987

40 PC OF TEENAGERS RUN RISK OF AIDS – SURVEY

Daily Telegraph, 24 July 1987.

Numerical estimates of Australians at risk from or already infected with HIV quoted in press accounts included '2 million Australians at risk . . . there are currently 50 000 carriers of the virus in Australia . . . one in 200 of sexually-active Australians carry the virus and can transmit it to others'. Such large figures reinforced the message that the disease had insidiously crept into Australian society-at-large and posed an awful threat to all Australians.

This quantification rhetoric ensured that AIDS was now presented as everybody's problem, for example in the following editorial:

Australia is faced with one of the gravest threats to the health of its people that it has ever confronted. No longer is AIDS a disease afflicting primarily homosexuals and drug addicts. It has broken through into the heterosexual community. It can now be picked up as easily as any other sexual disease. The difference is, it kills you. . . . Today there are at least 40 000 people walking around completely unaware they are AIDS antibody positive (in other words, they are carriers). The number will double every 10 months.

Sun Herald, 16 November 1986

As Potter, Wetherell and Chitty (1991) have pointed out, the use of quantification, although overtly a value-free product of mathematics, science and biomedicine, is, at the ideological level, a social construction deployed when proposing and undermining arguable cases. The way in which numerical values are used in the public health context is therefore revealing of powerful interests and subjective positions. The use to which quantification was put in press accounts dealing with AIDS risk offers an interesting example of the exploitation of numbers for such largely rhetorical purposes.

In press accounts of the threat posed by AIDS to Australians, as quoted above, the common use of quantification in concert with the suggestion that the majority of people infected with HIV were unaware that they were 'carriers', and predictions that these high figures were likely to increase rapidly, or even 'double every 10 months', implies certainty (because the figures are so precise). These discursive strategies also invoke apocalyptic imagery because of the claimed exponential nature of AIDS figures, denoting uncontrolled spread and disaster. This rhetoric dehumanizes by reducing asymptomatic people living with AIDS and those who are ill and dying to statistics. Ironically, however, such accounts suggested that these faceless statistics also posed a very human threat to others, as 'carriers' who may be unaware of their potential to transmit HIV infection. The implication of such quantification rhetoric was that AIDS was as easily transmissible as the common cold, as well as being as lethal as the plague, fuelling statements about the potential for mass loss of life. At the same time, the melodramatic use of quantification, in concert with the quoting of different figures in different accounts relating to the same phenomenon, may have served the purpose of inspiring disquiet while also creating confusion among members of the public as to their actual risk from HIV infection.

The end of the sexual revolution?

As noted earlier, from 1981 to 1985 articles on AIDS in the Australian press made frequent reference to the idea that AIDS was God's (or society's) retribution for the 'deviant' sexual behaviour of gay men (although not, it seems, of lesbians). In the 'Grim Reaper' years of AIDS reportage, the emphasis changed as the focus of press accounts of AIDS upon gay lifestyles diminished in favour of the threat posed by the disease to multi-partnered heterosexuals. The notion that fear of AIDS would occasion a return to 'old values', or to sexual and moral conservatism redolent of the Victorian era was often voiced in press articles referring to the disease. In late 1986, building up to the release of the 'Grim Reaper' campaign in early 1987, the print media began to refer to the change in sexual mores which would accompany the spread of the disease to heterosexuals. Expressive language used in these accounts focused upon the fundamental religious concerns of sex, death, punishment, divine retribution and sin as applied to permissive heterosexual activity.

Headlines such as,

CAUTION IS THE '80S WATCHWORD: AIDS AND THE WARTS VIRUS HAVE TAKEN OVER AS THE MAIN SEXUAL DANGERS
Time, 15 December 1986

and

A PERMISSIVE SOCIETY PAYS THE PRICE
Australian, 20 January 1987

began to appear in late 1986, suggesting that the new threat of AIDS to society was a consequence of permissive behaviour. The notion of deviance and deserved retribution apparent in press accounts thus widened to include all sexual behaviour not bonded by heterosexual monogamy. Articles suggested that sexual mores among heterosexuals were changing accordingly, as evidenced by the following headlines:

IT'S MUCH NICER SAYING NO: ROMANCE IS BACK IN FASHION ... NOW YOU LOVE TO BE WOOED
Sun, 1 July 1986

NEW MORALITY EMERGES IN SCANDINAVIA
Canberra Times, 16 December 1986

NEXT: NOT-SO-NAUGHTY NINETIES?
Courier-Mail, 8 December 1986

PROMISCUITY NOW A DIRTY WORD
Canberra Times, 18 March 1987

TIME TO TALK ABOUT MAKING MORALS RESPECTABLE AGAIN
Age, 31 March 1987

MALE VIRGINITY THE 'IN' THING
Daily Telegraph, 19 March 1987
MATRIMONY IS BACK IN FASHION: HERE COMES THE NEW MORALITY! RE-
TURN TO OLDTIME ATTITUDES IN LOVE, MARRIAGE AND SEX
Daily Mirror, 30 March 1987.

The message that casual sex was no longer acceptable came to dominate press accounts of AIDS. Ita Buttrose, as a quasi-religious leader,
contributed to this discourse by making public statements such as,
'casual sex is out, one-night stands are gone, multiple sex partners are
downright dangerous and so is sharing needles and syringes. The
sexual revolution is over' (*Launceston Examiner,* 6 April 1987). Articles
and headlines emphasized this theme in response to the release of
the 'Grim Reaper' campaign:

RETURN OF THE PRUDE? HERE COMES A NEW MORALITY
. . . The major social upheaval is down to one cause: AIDS. Outright fear of the fatal,
sexually transmitted disease has cast a black cloud over the sunny skies of free and
casual love affairs . . . If you won the right to say YES 20 years ago, today you can have
the right to say NO. Your life might depend on it.
News, 6 April 1987

BACK TO OLD VIRTUES
Daily Sun, 7 April 1987 [with photo of smiling bridal couple]

AIDS IS SAVING COUPLES
Fear of catching AIDS is keeping husbands and wives married, according to the
Institute of Family Studies. Researcher Margaret Harrison says the threat of the Grim
Reaper could save marriages, because people are less likely to have extra-marital
affairs.
Sun, 22 June 1987

According to an article published in the *Daily News* (9 April 1987),
accompanied by a photograph of the 'Grim Reaper', '[t]he 1990s
could become the decade of mass celibacy. A sexual revolution which
began in the 60s, gained momentum in the 70s and continued into
the 80s, could die a sudden death'. The remainder of the text went
on to predict widespread and dramatic social change, where 'Adam
and Eve would probably have an AIDS test before populating the
Garden of Eden'. The combination of the 'Grim Reaper' icon, Old
Testament references, the quoting of Buttrose's statements about the
demise of casual sex and the dramatic headline 'SEX ISN'T WORTH
DYING FOR' strongly oriented the article towards paternalistic moral
threats concerning punishment for permissive sexual expression.

This article was not alone in its warnings of punishment for sexual sinning. Editorials, in particular, suggested that AIDS was a warning signal to a society rendered dissolute by the excesses of the 1960s and 1970s. While on the one hand decrying sexual permissiveness, most editorials supported an explicitness in AIDS health education, declaring that the risk posed by AIDS was too great not to scare the sexually active into moral behaviour. The texts of the following editorials offer examples of this moralistic discourse which was such a common feature of AIDS reporting in the tabloid press (and to a lesser extent in 'quality' newspapers):

WHAT THE MIRROR SAYS: AIDS, SEX AND A NEW MORALITY

... One of the weapons we can use against AIDS is a dramatic change in our sex habits – a new morality, the cornerstone of which must be a re-examination of and a new responsibility in our sex lives. But mainly we can promote a return to fidelity and faithfulness and to the sanctity of marriage – three concepts that suffered in the promiscuous sixties ...

Daily Mirror, 30 March 1987

AIDS: COULD IT BE JUST THE JOLT WE NEED?

At an age when children once did not even know the facts of life, they are now being taught the potential terrors of a promiscuous life ... But isn't the truth about a decadent society being spelt out as well? Isn't it finally forcing us to face the fact that morally we've become a sick, sorry and seedy society ... Until recently, we would have poured scorn and derision on any clergyman preaching hell fire and that damnation is a consequence of evil. But perhaps that's exactly what's now needed. Because we *are* being damned by a terrible disease caused by unmitigated sexual lust.

Weekend Herald, December 13–14 1986

THE MORALITY OF AIDS

... Already the AIDS threat has prompted a real backlash to the free and easy sexual mores of the sixties and seventies. It is now time to recognize that every sexually active person has a duty to minimize the spread of the disease ... If it succeeds, the sexual clock will be turned back 20 years to before the promiscuous society and free love. The sad fact is, free love these days could be the kiss of death. Old-fashioned fidelity, with or without marriage, or no sex at all, is once again the way to stay out of trouble.

Advertiser, 26 March 1987

Many of the words and phrases used here hearken back to Biblical laws of fidelity and chastity, implying that those who transgress these edicts are to be punished for their sins: 'we are being damned by a terrible disease caused by unmitigated sexual lust'. Sexual activity is described as lacking responsibility, being 'sick, sorry and seedy', causing the 'backlash' of 'a terrible disease', constituting the 'kiss of death' and having 'potential terrors'. Such accounts repeat the simplistic notion that 'turning back the clock' to some golden mythical era of less promiscuity, decadence and 'unmitigated sexual lust' is the solution to the problem of AIDS. These accounts promote the moral message that old-fashioned religious values, chastity, fidelity and 'the sanctity of marriage' are the keys to protecting against AIDS. The metaphor 'AIDS is a moral reformer' emerges clearly here, as does 'Sex is dangerous', and 'AIDS is punishment' (for heterosexual, as well as homosexual, sexual activity). The overt meaning suggests that the one positive aspect of the AIDS epidemic is that casual sexual activity will cease by sheer necessity of survival. However, a closer examination of the rhetoric employed suggests that the hidden meaning may have been diametrically opposed. The words and noun phrases used to describe the 'new asexual revolution' are stodgy, plodding, Victorian and dull: 'wooed . . . morality . . . caution . . . not-so-naughty . . . respectable . . . curbs . . . old-time attitudes . . . prude . . . responsibility . . . fidelity . . . faithfulness . . . sanctity of marriage . . . safe . . . chaste . . . Biblical . . . old-fashioned . . . duty . . . no sex at all . . . stay out of trouble'. Here the press is taking on the role of the clergy, seeking to preach against sinful behaviour and to maintain conservative values. For the conservative reader, these moral lessons may well have struck the right chord. For the young and radical and sexually curious, however, the press' representation of sex in the time of AIDS may have appeared reactionary and stuffy, the voice of undesirable paternalism, with the effect of dismissing, amongst members of this subgroup, any intention to 'behave sensibly'. Such individuals would have read the meaning of the text in negotiated or oppositional ways. The words and phrases describing the behaviour likely to lead to AIDS: 'dirty word . . . promiscuity . . . danger . . . damned . . . free love . . . decadent . . . unmitigated sexual lust . . . free and easy sexual mores of the Sixties'; would appear attractively venial to some members of the audience, with 'the potential terrors of a promiscuous life' seeming a reward rather than a punishment.

Spotlight on condoms

Until the appearance of the 'Grim Reaper', condoms were unmentionable in polite society and rarely referred to in the press, even in 1986. However, once the focus of the press had turned to the heterosexual threat of AIDS, condoms were accorded the full glare of publicity and were the subject of several articles. The use of condoms to prevent against HIV infection became a matter of general discussion in the Australian press at the same time as the threat to heterosexuals of AIDS came on the public agenda – in late 1986, gaining momentum in early 1987. Articles were headlined with statements (and execrable puns) in support of condoms:

BETTER LATEX THAN NEVER

Times on Sunday, 8 March 1987

GIVE KIDS CONDOM MACHINES

Sunday Sun, 3 May 1987

CONDOM SALES UP

Daily Telegraph, 15 February 1988

CONDOM ADS HERALD NEW TV ERA

Australian, 27 March 1987

CONDOM BILLED AS SHEER DELIGHT

Advertiser, 10 February 1987.

Many editorials and feature articles endorsed the recommendations of public health officials that condoms be brought out of the closet and into public discourse. One editorial in the *Advertiser* (23 March 1987), for example, was approving of the Australian government's stance on condom use, remarking that '... in the light of present knowledge about AIDS, and the general benefit to the community, the Government is doing the right thing'. Other newspapers thoughtfully provided user's guides to condoms, alleging that 'Australia's most maligned contraceptive – for generations the butt of jokes about dingers, frangers, rubbers and raincoats – the condom has finally become respectable' (*Times on Sunday*, 10 May 1987). The condom was described favourably as having had 'a dizzying rise in social status' and as 'an instrument of national salvation' by the *Newcastle Herald* (13 February 1987). Condoms were compared favourably with biomedical treatments and medical technology, thus gaining respectability by association. The *Financial Review* (17 February 1987) spoke of 'the extraordinary metamorphosis of the condom' into an object imbued by the medical profession with 'medical significance on a par with the discovery of penicillin or the Salk vaccine'. Such representations of condoms drew upon several metaphors relating to condoms, including 'Condom as lifesaver', 'Condom as saviour of humankind', and 'Condom as protector'. Several features made the suggestion that an insistence upon condoms could represent a way for women to take control in their sexual relationships, invoking the metaphors 'Condom as control' and 'Condom as feminist power'. Several newspapers, including the *Hobart Mercury* (14 January 1987) quoted Ita Buttrose as asserting that 'now it was up to women to take a stand by practising safe sex, particularly by insisting on the use of condoms'. An article entitled 'SEX AND THE SMART GIRL' (*Launceston Sunday Examiner*,

15 February 1987) made the same point, as did another which raised the metaphor 'condom as fashion item':

> Today's thinking girl has them neatly filed in her cosmetics case ... says 20-year old fashion student, Katie Grove: 'I always carry a condom. It's no longer a matter of shame or embarrassment that you run around with one in your handbag. In fact, it's almost trendy to be seen carrying them'.
>
> *Daily News*, 24 July 1987

Related to this metaphor, and also drawing upon the metaphor 'condom as product,' the financial possibilities offered by the fear of AIDS received major attention in the business pages of newspapers. The condom was presented as an everyday commodity which now was advertised commercially and bought at boutiques, record shops and supermarkets. The fashion aspect of the devices was discussed by the *Advertiser* (10 February 1987), which reported them as being packaged in a 'stylish little box', and the *Launceston Sunday Examiner* (15 February 1987), which noted that condoms were being marketed to appeal to women in 'slim-line packs in pastel shades'.

Not all press accounts about condoms in the age of AIDS were positive, however. Some headlines reflected the controversial nature of the topic:

BISHOPS CONDEMN 'CONDOM CULTURE'
Herald, 20 May 1987

MORAL QUANDARIES AND CONDOMS
Times on Sunday, 15 February 1987

CONDOM FEAR FOR KIDS
Sun, 14 April 1987

ROW FLARES ON CONDOM ITEM
News, 29 July 1987

STUDENTS TAUNT POLICE OVER CONDOM MACHINES
Daily Sun, 25 July 1987

LIBERAL MP OPPOSES CONDOMS IN CLASS
West Australian, 28 April 1987.

As these headlines imply, conservative politicians, lobbyists and the clergy were in the forefront of outrage about the sudden rise to acclaim of the condom, and their comments received wide coverage in the press. The words 'oppose ... condemn ... fear ... row ... flares ... taunt' suggest divisiveness and conflict, and imply that condoms were still not widely acceptable in Australian society.

The condom continued to attract controversy throughout the 'Grim Reaper' period of AIDS reporting. The Queensland state government was beset by a highly publicized controversy about the promotion of condoms as prophylactics which began to receive much attention in the press in July 1987, staying an issue for several months. A right-wing Member of the Western Australian State Parliament was quoted as asserting that introducing information into West Australian schools was not the answer to combating AIDS, for 'If young students are going to be encouraged to feel, stretch and handle condoms, then I leave it to you to work out what the next step will be' (*West Australian*, 28 April 1987). The upper echelons of the Catholic Church in Australia were quoted as stating that 'We reject any form of education which relies on a single-minded promotion of prophylactics and fails to present moral responsibility and chastity as the true and best remedy' (*Herald*, 20 May 1987). One article (*Times on Sunday*, 15 February 1987) opined that 'under no circumstances will the Catholic Church in Australia advocate publicly that homosexuals should use condoms', for according to a Church spokesman, 'whether they do it with or without a condom, it's the same act. If someone commits murder, it's morally irrelevant that they stole the axe'. The recurrence of tropes linking condoms to impiety, promiscuity, immorality and homosexuality highlighted the controversial nature of condoms and drew upon older and more well-established meanings surrounding them.

Condoms also received negative publicity by association with male-to-male sexual activities in jails. A continuing area of controversy which has received much attention in the Australian press is that of the distribution of condoms in jails. Despite the repeated urging of health officials that condoms be freely handed out to prisoners so that they might avoid spreading HIV by anal intercourse, some State politicians had difficulty accepting that men in prisons engage in male-to-male sexual practices. One politician was widely quoted in the press as saying 'I don't see any need for us to issue condoms. After all, homosexuality is illegal in Queensland' (*Courier-Mail*, 18 May 1987). Headlines about this controversial topic included:

PLEA FOR SALE OF CONDOMS TO PRISONERS

Daily Sun, 15 May 1987

PRISONS MAY SELL CONDOMS

Canberra Times, 16 May 1987

CONDOMS WON'T BE ISSUED IN QLD JAILS

Canberra Times, 18 May 1987.

According to the *Sun Herald* (1 November 1987), warders at Bathurst Jail refused to distribute government-issued condoms to the prisons because, in the view of one warder, 'Bathurst would be known as the "homo jail of Australia". It is not fair on the blokes who work there, or the prisoners'. Condoms in this context thus became symbols of triple deviance: crime, AIDS and homosexual activities.

The relative reliability of condoms was the object of much discussion in the print media in 1987, reflecting the concurrent debate in the medical literature about the effectiveness of condoms as a barrier against HIV. Articles reported complaints from users about condoms easily breaking (*Sun*, 7 May 1987). Such reports provided a voice of dissent to the confident predictions that the promotion of condom use was the solution to AIDS, and was seized upon by moralists as a good reason to adopt chastity and monogamy rather than rely upon condoms. For example, an Anglican Archbishop was reported as saying that 'people had to realize that condoms were not a guarantee of immunity against the disease ... It should be noted that Christian moral obligations in sexual relationships are the best health provisions' (*Courier-Mail*, 9 November 1987).

To summarize, recurring phrases and assertions about condoms which were positive included the following: condoms are safeguards, lifesavers; condoms are a source of wealth, present an entrepreneurial opportunity to shrewd businesspeople; condoms are a good weapon against AIDS, combat AIDS, provide defence against AIDS; condoms provide a responsible, mature way to have sex, a new way of loving; condoms are reliable; condoms protect against other sexually transmissible diseases and are contraceptives with no side-effects; condoms provide a way for women to assert themselves and take the initiative; using condoms is a humorous, novel, fun way to have sex; the condom is now a household word, is respectable, just another consumer product on supermarket shelves; condoms are a smart accessory for men and women on the go, are smart sex.

However, negative phrases and assertions often appearing in press accounts were also numerous, including the following: condom sizes are a source of embarrassment to men; the promotion of condoms encourage promiscuity, spread the message of free sex; used condoms pollute the environment; condoms have a high failure rate, give a false sense of security, give no guarantee; condoms have no place in true love or romance; condoms smell of rubber, are unnatural, sex with condoms is not the real thing; using condoms spoils spontaneity, is a passion killer, dampens the libido; condoms are a big joke, are not serious, are embarrassing, are silly little pieces of rubber; condom use is against Christian belief; condoms encourage homosexuality; condom is a dirty word, is offensive; condom use encourages lack of self-control; talking about condoms in schools encourages sexual behaviour in school children; condoms are used by prostitutes, are seedy, promote marital infidelity, are indecent; condoms are used by fumbling teenage boys.

These lists drawn from press accounts of condoms during this middle period of AIDS reporting demonstrate that despite AIDS educators' desire to popularize condom use, the messages transmitted about condoms in the newspaper reports were diverse, contradictory and included many negative conceptualizations. Given that these contradictions were expressed in the popular press, there is reason to suggest that the failure of members of the general population to embrace the use of condoms may partly result from the diverse meanings communicated to them in this forum.

The personalization of AIDS risk

A key discursive strategy used in the press during the 'Grim Reaper' period of AIDS reporting to bring the threat of AIDS closer to its readers was to 'personalize' accounts, or to present a story from the point of view of one 'ordinary' person, who, it was suggested, is just like 'you and me'. As Fowler (1991: 92) suggests, the technique of personalization serves to make an issue more concrete, especially if personal details such as age, residence, occupation and physical appearance are given, with the liberal use of photographs. Individuals are categorized and reduced to stereotypes by this process.

In one example of the use of personalization in press accounts of AIDS, a journalist wrote a 'personal point-of-view' article about having an HIV antibody test. In his account, the use of categorization is evident. He is careful to emphasize that he is not gay, or an injecting drug user, or a man who sees prostitutes: he is just an 'ordinary guy', and belonging to that new at-risk category makes him a 'candidate' for HIV infection. However, the point of the story is that the journalist himself, despite belonging to none of these supposedly deviant groups, is still at risk of infection. The old stigmatized stereotypes are carefully maintained, but are replaced with a new one – the young, white-collar male at risk from HIV infection through heterosexual sexual activity:

PUTTING THE AIDS TEST TO THE TEST

Suddenly all the jokes aren't so funny. Sitting in a waiting room minutes away from an AIDS test, I feel uncomfortable ... It's ridiculous, but I try not to look gay, I try not to look like an intravenous drug user and I try not to look like I've been with a prostitute. They are the ones who end up with AIDS. Not me – I'm an ordinary guy. But I can't be sure I'm clear. The simple fact that I am an ordinary guy makes me a candidate. It means that I've experienced the 'casual encounters'. And that I didn't always wear a condom.

Herald, 13 April 1987

This personalized account is unusual not only because it was written from the point of view of the journalist, turning a usually 'objective' voice into one which is 'subjective' and humanized, but because the person concerned is male. During this period of reporting, nearly all other personalized accounts of people at risk of HIV infection, or already infected, were about young *women*. The articles excerpted below offer examples of this more general patterning:

HOW AIDS THREATENS ALL OF US

Joanna's case is a fairly typical one. When Joanna went to university she was confident that a stable home background and a high school education would ensure a stimulating social life and a reasonably good degree . . . When she realized that survival for two years after the first attack of *Pneumocystis carinii* is, at its best, very rare, and that she would never experience either marriage or children, she attempted suicide. Cases like this are still a rarity. If the disease is allowed to spread, they will become commonplace.

Sun Herald, 23 November 1986

WOMEN AT RISK CAN AVOID VIRUS

Alison never had sex with anyone except her husband. Last year she was one of 17 women in Britain who died from AIDS. She did not know her husband was bisexual . . . Only one case of heterosexual transmission of AIDS, from man to woman, has been detected in Queensland. But State health officials say married or promiscuous women are at greater risk from the virus than prostitutes, who are tested every three months. They are at risk mainly from bisexual men who pass on the disease.

Daily Sun, 4 March 1987

BRAVE VICTIM FIGHTS TO LIVE

. . . Sarah caught AIDS from a man she fell in love with in Australia. Chris was handsome, successful and charming. Their future together was taking shape. Everything seemed ideal. But Chris was bi-sexual. He was the third man with whom young Sarah had made love and she had no way of knowing . . . [She said] 'Several girls I have met with AIDS have got it from bi-sexual men. How exactly are you supposed to tell? And make no mistake there are all sorts of myths about it like you have to have prolonged exposure or you get it because you are promiscuous. Actually you can get it the first time you make love, just as you can get pregnant the first time'.

Daily News, 2 April 1987

SHE'S DYING OF AIDS: BUT IT WASN'T HER FAULT SHE FELL FOR THE WRONG GUY

No one told secretary Sunnye Sherman that she could catch AIDS at home in her own bed, from the man she was engaged to marry. Yet she is living and dying proof that you don't have to be a drug addict, prostitute, homosexual or even receive blood transfusions to catch the killer disease.

Sunday Territorian, 27 July 1986

These stories about women with AIDS were sometimes accompanied by before and after photographs, the before portrait showing the subject smiling and pretty, the after shot showing her looking wan, ill and thin, gazing pensively at the camera. This usage of the before and after shot has been described by Crimp (1992: 129) as a 'standard media device for constructing AIDS as a morality tale', and is routinely used in documentaries about gay people living with AIDS. The stories are remarkably similar in many respects: the women are portrayed as innocent and unfortunate victims, who were blameless and unsuspecting of the risk they were taking in having sex with their male partners: 'it wasn't her fault she fell for the wrong guy . . . she had no way of knowing . . . she did not know that her husband was bisexual . . . How exactly are you supposed to tell?'. The women epitomize normal, white, middle-class, fun-living heterosexuals who were allegedly the vanguard of the new breed of AIDS victims. Their 'ordinariness' is emphasized in their stories: Sunnye, for example, is 'living and dying proof that you don't have to be a drug addict, prostitute, homosexual or even receive blood transfusions to catch the killer disease', while Joanna's case is 'a fairly typical one'.

The relationships concerned are painted in a rosy, romantic light, echoing the genre of romantic women's fiction: for example, 'Chris was handsome, successful and charming. Their future together was taking shape. Everything seemed ideal . . .', or as a harmless and understandable peccadillo of youthful sexual experimenting, 'as part of final year joie de vivre'. It is emphasized in these accounts that the women were not sexually promiscuous, but rather, unlucky in their trust in their sexual partner: Alison 'never had sex with anyone but her husband', while Sunnye contracted HIV from 'the man she was engaged to marry'. In most cases, the partner was discovered (too late) to be bisexual, and the apparent 'normality' of the relationship was exposed as a pretence.

With the proliferation of such personalized accounts, the archetype of the AIDS 'victim' had changed from the gay man or (less frequently) the person with haemophilia and the injecting drug user to the innocent young heterosexual girl or faithful married woman at the mercy of male promiscuity. The moral of these stories is clear: if you are a heterosexual woman, do not trust your partners, for you are now at risk of death: 'Cases like this are still a rarity. If the disease is allowed to spread they will become commonplace'. Given the assertion that the stories were highly relevant to Australian audiences, it is interesting to note that the majority of these moral tales were in fact syndicated from foreign newspapers, being about women resident in countries other than Australia (for example, Sunnye and Joanna were American, Alison was British). Even when it was admitted that similar cases are currently rare in Australia: 'Only one case of heterosexual transmission of AIDS, from man to woman, has been detected in Queensland', the *potential* of the threat posed to 'ordinary' women was emphasized: '. . . married or promiscuous women are at greater risk from the virus than prostitutes, who are tested every three months. They are at risk mainly from bisexual men who pass on the disease'. Similar stories presenting heterosexual men as vulnerable to acquiring HIV infection from women were few.

'Suzi's Story'

News media interest in personalizing news stories about heterosexuals contracting HIV reached its apotheosis when a documentary entitled 'Suzi's Story', was screened on Australian commercial television about the death from AIDS of an heterosexual woman living in Sydney, Suzi Lovegrove. Although Suzi was American by birth and had contracted HIV in New York before moving to Australia, her story was presented as a tragic example of an Australian woman with AIDS. In June 1987, following closely upon the heels of the 'Grim Reaper' campaign, the story of Suzi's death presented an opportunity to bring home the threat of AIDS to heterosexuals. The documentary received much publicity in the Australian press, with most articles about her story being accompanied by wedding photos of Suzi, an attractive woman in her early thirties, accompanied by her husband. In such photographs, both gaze at the camera with open, attractive and 'ordinary' smiles. Their smiles contrast cruelly with the headlines and captions: 'TV viewers will watch Suzi die . . . AIDS tragedy is set to shock . . . Dancer and choreographer Suzi Lovegrove . . . tragic end to a young life . . . family shattered'.

Suzi, according to news reports, had caught HIV before meeting her husband from a casual affair with a man she later discovered was bisexual. Like the stories of the women described above, Suzi was thus an unsuspecting victim of AIDS, who did not deserve her fate. By the time AIDS was diagnosed, Suzi had married and given birth to a son, who was also diagnosed HIV antibody positive. She and her husband agreed to allow a television crew to film her in the closing stages of her illness, as an educative measure for other heterosexuals. The documentary had great dramatic power: the combination of a young and attractive woman, happily married with a baby son but dying painfully of AIDS, was the kind of tragic story beloved by the press. Reports of Suzi's death in June 1987 were accompanied by photographs of her toddler son at the funeral. Headlines about Suzi's case emphasized the tragedy, her courage and the lesson it posed for others:

TRAGIC SUZI'S FIGHT FOR LIFE: A HARROWING LOOK AT AIDS
Daily Mirror, 17 June 1987
ANGUISH AND TORMENT FOR VICTIM SUZI: AIDS TRAGEDY SHOCKS
News, 18 June 1987
TRAGEDY TO SHATTER APATHY OVER AIDS
Daily Telegraph, 23 June 1987
SUZI'S STORY OF COURAGE
Daily Sun, 25 June 1987.

Feature articles were explicit in presenting Suzi's case as a parable of modern times which should warn others of the possible consequences of careless sexual activity:

> Having a casual affair should not mean a sentence to the casualty ward, but too often it does. Such a casual affair not only ruined but took the life of a young New York dancer and choreographer ... Suzi permitted a film crew to put the final three months of her life on tape in a bid to make the community aware of the disease and to prove it is not only a disease which threatens homosexuals or those who are promiscuous.
>
> *Daily Telegraph,* 23 June 1987

Suzi Lovegrove's illness and death from AIDS and the circumstances in which she had become infected offered a convenient real-life example of NACAIDS' warnings that casual heterosexual activity can lead to an early painful and tragic death, filled with 'torment' and 'anguish'. Once again, reports emphasized the unlucky circumstances of her infection with HIV, the fact that she had 'no way of knowing' that she was at risk, that Suzi 'was not an intravenous drug user. She was not promiscuous', that a casual affair can ruin and take lives, that AIDS 'is now very much a heterosexual disease' and 'can no longer be classed as a gay plague' (*Sunday Telegraph,* 21 June 1987). Even 'true love', a happy marriage and loving husband had not protected Suzi from the disease (*Sun,* 23 June 1987).

It is worthy of note that Suzi Lovegrove, like the other heterosexual women whose stories were personalized by the press, was positioned as an 'innocent victim' of AIDS who had not deserved her fate, and whose illness and death was a terrible tragedy, said to prove that AIDS is 'not only a disease which threatens homosexuals or those who are promiscuous'. No other people living with AIDS who died during the 'Grim Reaper' period of AIDS reporting occasioned the press attention and sympathy accorded Suzi. Although many 'ordinary' gay men died of AIDS between July 1986 and June 1988, none were publicly mourned in the Australian press. The story provided ballast for the assertions of NACAIDS that Australian heterosexuals were now at risk, and that complacency was dangerous, adding timely publicity to the message of the 'Grim Reaper' campaign. For example, Ita Buttrose was reported as remarking that 'What [Suzi Lovegrove] has shown is that a heterosexual woman can get AIDS just as easily as a homosexual. The fact that she got it from a casual affair enforces NACAIDS' view that one-night stands are out' (*West Australian*, 24 June 1987).

Dissenting voices

It would be misleading to give the impression that the Australian press was uniformly consistent in supporting the state's stand on AIDS education and policy. In fact there were several instances during the 'Grim Reaper' period of AIDS reporting in which the dominant AIDS discourses were challenged. Challenges came from a number of prominent individuals and groups who refused to acknowledge that AIDS was quite the threat to heterosexuals it had been made out to be. For example, moral conservatives were reported as being opposed to the 'Grim Reaper' advertizements because they detracted attention from gay men and injecting drug users. The Reverend Fred Nile, a member of the New South Wales Parliament and leader of the Christian fundamentalist movement the Festival of Light, was quoted as being very concerned that they did not 'address those in the high risk categories', and asking 'The star is a crying, frightened six-year-old girl. How is the little girl going to get AIDS? Does she have a sexual partner?' (*Illawarra Mercury*, 7 April 1987). Another conservative politician was reported as saying that the advertizement 'unfairly engendered a pervasive atmosphere of suspicion and distrust by implying that everyone risks exposure to the virus through sexual contact' (*Launceston Examiner*, 6 April 1987). Yet another politician was quoted as saying that the campaign was 'hypocritical because the Federal government has actively promoted the destructive, dangerous and degrading homosexual lifestyle' (*Launceston Examiner*, April 11, 1987).

The letters to the editor section of newspapers is one of the few forums in the mass media where 'ordinary' people are provided the opportunity to freely express their opinions on current events unmediated by journalists' reframing (talk-back radio is another). The release of the 'Grim Reaper' campaign proved to be inspiring for letter writers, for the newspaper letter pages in April 1987 were dominated by heated debates concerning the campaign. It is interesting to note that while editorials and articles were largely supportive of the campaign, letter writers expressed a number of objections about the style and substance of the advertizements. Some letter writers commented that the introduction of the 'Grim Reaper' would 'reinforce people's fear of death and dying rather than be identified with the more specific threat of AIDS' (*Advertiser*, 14 April 1987); 'I worry about death being depicted as a terrifying Grim Reaper. We are trying to encourage people to accept death calmly and without fear, and this medieval concept is unnecessary and insensitive' (*Australian*, 15 April 1987). One woman asked, 'How many people are watching loved ones die, or are dying themselves (from whatever cause) are led to unnecessary fear through that dreadful portrayal of death as a grim (and mocking) reaper? (*Australian*, 14 April 1987).

Several letter writers made the point that the use of fear in health education was likely to be counterproductive. One writer to the *Age* (7 April 1987) opined that 'Scare tactics don't work, they reinforce the "it will never happen to me" attitude'. The head of an educational development and research institute wrote to express his alarm at the use of fear in the campaign, for 'Behaviour modification programmes based on accurate information are most effective; programmes based on fear show a mixture of unfortunate side-effects and consequences' (*Age*, 18 April 1987). Another letter writer commented, '. . . the advertisement has such horrifying images, who will listen to any message? My young children are so terrified we have to switch it off' (*Age*, 7 April 1987). One exasperated reader wrote to the editor of the *Daily Telegraph*: 'I don't know if I will ever get sick from AIDS, but by God I'm sick of hearing about it!' (22 April 1987).

In serving the claim to free speech and in the interests of inciting controversy, homophobic attitudes received expression more overtly in this section than in other sections of newspapers. The fact that gay men were the first to contract HIV in large numbers was mentioned by several writers, often in a negative light. It was asserted that gay or bisexual men were still those at most risk of contracting HIV: 'While it is acknowledged that AIDS is now widespread in the heterosexual community, initially, women in this country . . . appear to have become the victims of sexually deviant males who hop into bed with wives or girlfriends after sexual sessions with other males' (*Australian*,

14 April 1987). The depiction of a mother with babe-in-arms and a little girl as victims of the bowling ball inspired the criticism that such individuals were not at risk from HIV: 'AIDS is being presented as a disease which women catch from men, its most prominent advertised "victims" being a young girl, and a mother and child. In fact, the victims of AIDS in this country have almost all been homosexual men' (*Age*, 12 April 1987): 'Why spend millions of dollars frightening millions of people when a much lesser amount spent educating the minority groups who are responsible for the disease could be far more effective in eradicating it?' (*Launceston Examiner*, 14 April 1987). The campaign were seen as promoting permissiveness: 'I am still waiting for Bob Hawke [Prime Minister at the time] to tell us who gave his government permission to encourage a permissive society' (*Australian*, 14 April 1987); but also as creating anxiety about sexuality: '. . . the highly emotive content of the campaign leaves me wondering about its motivation. We will have to guard against this approach leading to prejudice against the victims and a paranoia against sexuality in general' (*Age*, 7 April 1987). Not all letters, however, were negative. Several lauded the campaign, commenting on its effectiveness. For example, a writer to the *West Australian* (11 April 1987) commented that 'such shock treatment should be praised, not condemned', while a letter published in the *Daily Sun* (27 April 1987) said, 'Congratulations to the Federal Government, you have shocked us into the reality of AIDS. To the people who complain about this ad, you are just plain ignorant'.

Apart from letter writers, objections to the 'Grim Reaper' campaign reproduced in newspaper accounts were largely voiced by moralists and ultra-conservative politicians, who unlike Britain and the USA have limited power in Australian society. Such dissent, couched as it was in overtly discriminatory language, could largely be discounted as prejudiced rather than arising from considered opinions. In terms of sheer volume, dissenting views collectively constituted a small voice against the prevailing support given by the press to the government's AIDS policy and decision to launch the 'Grim Reaper' campaign. It seemed as if the agenda had been set by the dramatic and highly newsworthy messages and imagery employed in the 'Grim Reaper' campaign and its promotion, and attempts at this stage in the history of AIDS reporting to counter the newsworthy story of AIDS as an apocalyptic threat to everyone received little attention.

Statements of dissent made by one anointed 'AIDS expert', Professor David Penington, however, did receive wide publicity because of his elite status as a professor and eminent physician, and his leading role in government AIDS organizations. Penington, a widely acknowledged authority on AIDS, had been involved with AIDS policy from the start of the epidemic and was able to supply a scholarly medical 'expert' opinion on the issue. Although initially publicly warning of the risk of HIV infection among multi-partnered heterosexuals, Penington was later to criticize the content of the 'Grim Reaper' campaign. His criticism was the subject of several articles and headlines:

ADS INDULGE IN OVERKILL: FORCE

The AIDS television campaign indulged in overkill by saying all promiscuous Australians had the same risk of contracting the disease, the National AIDS Task Force chairman, Professor David Penington, said yesterday. Professor Penington said promiscuous heterosexuals had 100 times less chance of getting AIDS than homosexuals and much less chance than intravenous drug users. This was because more homosexuals now had AIDS and practised anal sex more frequently.

Courier-Mail, 8 April 1987

AIDS NOW AFFECTS 17 500 AUSTRALIANS: PENINGTON

The number of Australians infected with the AIDS virus has reached 17 500, but only 20 acquired their disease through heterosexual transmission, a study released yesterday claims. The head of the AIDS Task Force, Professor David Penington, who released the study, used the figures to make his clearest statement yet that AIDS is only a heterosexual disease in exceptional circumstances ... Professor Penington specifically countered claims made by the Federal Government in its Grim Reaper campaign. 'It's not fair to say the disease is frequent in the community, that everybody is at equal risk or that anybody who has had more than one heterosexual partner is at risk in the same way as people who have engaged in intravenous drug abuse or male homosexual anal intercourse,' he said.

Australian, 14 May 1987

Several articles about AIDS in late 1987 were devoted to the dispute between Penington and NACAIDS, and questioned whether the risk to heterosexuals was real or inflated. Penington, however, was almost a lone voice amongst 'AIDS experts' in questioning NACAIDS' strategies and public statements about the risks posed by AIDS to heterosexuals, and lack of support from other quarters eroded his influence as a news actor in shaping discourses on AIDS. Penington later resigned from the AIDS Taskforce, and his high publicity profile as news actor was taken over by Dr Julian Gold, Director of the Albion Street AIDS Clinic, and Professor John Dwyer, an immunologist from the University of New South Wales, both of whom supported NACAIDS' endeavours.

Concurrent with the above debate, the odd article was published reporting the findings of research indicating that perhaps heterosexuals were not as at risk from AIDS to the extent stated by NACAIDS; for example:

REAPER'S SMALL TOLL

Only two of 6000 AIDS blood tests conducted since the Grim Reaper campaign started four weeks ago have proved positive, an AIDS expert said today. The results confirm doctors' beliefs that the deadly virus has not yet spread widely beyond homosexuals and drug users, says Dr Ian Gust, of Melbourne's Fairfield Hospital.

Sun, 5 May 1987

SCIENTISTS CALCULATE LONG ODDS ON WOMEN CATCHING AIDS

A woman's odds of catching AIDS from a single sexual encounter with an infected man are about one in 1000, says a report presented yesterday to the Third International Conference on AIDS in Washington.

Weekend Australian, 6–7 June 1987

AIDS RISK LOW FOR WOMEN

A study of AIDS-infected men and their female sex partners shows the virus is far less infectious to heterosexuals than once thought.

Daily Sun, 15 August 1987

These accounts provided a counterweight against the florid excesses of the majority of articles about the potential rapid spread of AIDS amongst heterosexuals, which, as noted above, tended to use melodramatic rhetoric and cite impossibly large numbers to make the case that AIDS poses a threat to all. In several dissenting accounts, quantification rhetoric was used to counter hyperbolic claims that AIDS was threatening millions of Australians, but did so in a manner which was equally confusing because of the different probabilities cited; examples from articles include the statement 'promiscuous heterosexuals ha[ve] 100 times less chance of getting AIDS than homosexuals' versus the assertion that 'a woman's odds of catching AIDS from a single sexual encounter with an infected man are about one in 1000'.

Why was there not more dissent from moralistic, religious, medical or scientific quarters about the extreme statements of risk made by Buttrose and Blewett during the 'Grim Reaper' period of AIDS reporting? One reason for the lack of reporting of dissenting opinion was the felicitous choice of Buttrose as head of NACAIDS, a person with immense media clout and public credibility. Other reasons may be related to the real sense of crisis felt by the Australian government about the threat of AIDS which was effectively communicated to the press, and the subsequent unwillingness of people in prominent positions to challenge the assertions of NACAIDS and risk a political backlash. Aspects related to the principles of newsworthiness may also have prevailed against a more balanced and cautious coverage of the threat posed by AIDS to heterosexuals, including the sheer dramatic value of the story, the steady stream of news items wired from news agencies in the USA and Britain which had the same themes of 'apocalypse now', and the unwillingness of journalists to enter into a debate which required a sophisticated understanding of epidemiology and biomedicine, and which was yet to be clearly defined in the medical literature in a format which could be easily translated to the audience. Within the formulae and lexicon of discourses on AIDS in the press during this period, it would have been difficult to accommodate more moderate or dissenting views.

Diminishing interest in heterosexuals and AIDS

It was inevitable that media attention to heterosexual risk would diminish given the lack of new issues or events to keep the story alive. The spotlight of attention which had been directed at heterosexuals and their risk of contracting HIV through casual sexual intercourse was beginning to dim by the end of 1987 because of lack of new stories. This diminishing interest was accompanied by a fall in the number of articles about AIDS printed in the Australian press, although there was a brief sharp rise in articles in November 1987, in which the new major topics were the burying of a car by police in which a man who had AIDS was killed, the order by a USA court that singer David Bowie submit to an HIV antibody test after an allegation of rape was brought against him, and the announcement that a message about safer sex was to be included on pornographic video tapes sold in Australia. As earlier shown in Figure 4.1, the numbers of articles about AIDS dropped dramatically towards the end of 1987. After December 1987, a slow news month for AIDS, the numbers of AIDS articles returned to pre-'Grim Reaper' levels. The intensity of coverage did not increase significantly in the first six months of 1988: in the first two quarters of that year, only 1965 AIDS items were published in the press, compared with 3440 during the same period in 1987.

However in early 1988 press interest in the heterosexual AIDS epidemic was temporarily invigorated by the publication of a monograph by the renowned sex researchers William Masters and Virginia Johnson (collaborating with Robert Kolodny). The book was entitled *Crisis: Heterosexual Behaviour in the Age of AIDS*, with the subheading 'This Book Could Save Your Life'. The authors' extreme statements concerning the transmissibility of HIV, including the claim that it was possible to catch the virus from mosquitoes, eating utensils and lavatory seats, caused controversy and renewed panic statements in the press. The *Australian* printed excerpts from their book under the headline

EPIDEMIC: A DISEASE RUNS WILD

with the subheading 'Heterosexuals are in danger: misinformation about AIDS is plunging them towards a formidable death toll' (7 March 1988). The first page of this article quoted large sections from the more extreme and apocalyptic statements made by Masters, Johnson and Kolodny in their book, including: 'AIDS is breaking out. The AIDS virus is now running rampant in the heterosexual community. Unless something is done to contain this global epidemic, we face a mounting death toll in the years ahead that will be the most formidable the world has ever seen'.

Such statements, reproduced verbatim with virtually no critical comment, served to promote the book as well as attracting sales of the newspaper. Other newspapers similarly quoted from the book uncritically, with such headlines as

MASTERS AND JOHNSON SOCK AN AIDS WARNING TO MULTI-PARTNER HETEROS

and quoted Masters as saying 'We've established a new high-risk group – the multi-partner heterosexual' (*Hobart Mercury*, 11 March 1988). These initial reports were however later countered by articles which reported criticisms of Masters, Johnson and Kolodny's work. The *Advertiser* (12 March 1988), for example, noted that 'The National Advisory Committee on AIDS yesterday criticized the controversial Masters and Johnson survey issue last week which claimed AIDS was rampant in the heterosexual community'. Such conflicting statements, in concert with reference to disparate probabilities of contracting HIV and varying estimates to the numbers of Australians at risk from AIDS in press accounts, may have continued to promote confusion amongst readers as to the reality of the threat.

As can be seen in the list of major topics presented in Appendix 2, press coverage in the first six months of 1988, apart from the flurry of attention paid to heterosexuals and AIDS in the wake of publication of Masters, Johnson and Kolodny's book, returned to a primary focus upon the bizarre and the biomedical. Coverage became more pluralistic and less dramatic. The emphasis of articles moved from personalizing the threat of AIDS to heterosexuals to reporting incidents involving royalty and Hollywood film stars: for example, Princess Anne made a discriminatory comment about people living with AIDS at an AIDS conference, Elizabeth Taylor's daughter-in-law was found to have AIDS, a friend of Princess Margaret was reported to have AIDS and a famous pornographic actor died of AIDS. During the first half of 1988 such bizarre incidents made headlines as an HIV antibody positive soccer referee being charged by the British Football Association with bringing the game into disrepute, the uncovering of a conspiracy to kidnap a Sydney businessman's teenage son and to threaten to inject him with HIV-infected blood, an Australian academic suggesting that HIV-infected people should be paid to forego sex to prevent HIV transmission and an elderly Australian couple contracting HIV. Less attention was paid to the use of health education as a 'weapon' against AIDS during the first six months of 1988. Medical advances related to AIDS again received attention. The preliminary results of AZT drug trials in Australia were reported in May 1988, and the first overseas clinical trials on humans of a possible vaccine was announced the following month, as was the development of a saliva test for antibodies to HIV.

In 1988 there was a greater emphasis upon injecting drug users as a group at increased risk of AIDS compared with reporting in 1987, when the focus upon heterosexual behaviour and AIDS risk overshadowed the risk posed by injecting drug use. In February 1988 it was suggested in some press accounts that injecting drug users would cause the 'second wave' of the AIDS epidemic. By June 1988 the National Health and Medical Council was reported as making the controversial suggestion that heroin users be given heroin to stop them sharing needles, and thereby decreasing their risk of contracting HIV. The AIDS in prisons issue also began to attract extensive coverage from October 1987 when five prisoners died in a fire deliberately started in Pentridge Jail as a protest about arrangements concerning HIV-infected prisoners. AIDS in prisons continued to be newsworthy into early 1988, largely fuelled by Professor John Dwyer's warnings in January 1988 that an AIDS crisis loomed in these institutions.

Summary

The 'Grim Reaper' AIDS education campaign, although run for only six weeks in April and May 1987, captured an extraordinary amount of media attention. It seemed that the ghost of the 'Gay Plague' had been laid by the coverage of the 'Grim Reaper' campaign, for press accounts no longer centred on this representation of AIDS, and gay men received little attention in press accounts. AIDS metaphors sought to generalize the disease, to show that all 'promiscuous' sex was dangerous and punishable by death, to 'shock the general population out of its complacency'. AIDS became a disease of 'self', rather than of the 'other'. Accompanying this shift in focus was an increased emphasis upon the negative aspects of heterosexual promiscuity, in which the representation of young women as the new 'victims' of AIDS dominated, but the heterosexual male 'victim' was rarely identified.

In press accounts, the government was positioned metaphorically as a paternal and disciplinary figure, seeking to disseminate knowledge which in turn would enjoin the masses to take responsibility for their own health. The press thus largely supported the government's attempts to impose a 'new morality', demonstrating its inherent conservativeness. However, the attention accorded by the press to the threat of AIDS to heterosexuals had begun to diminish by late 1987 and early 1988. News about the AIDS risk to heterosexuals was no longer fresh and exciting, and it had become more and more difficult to find a different 'angle' on stories about AIDS, or to maintain the aura of panic about the threats posed by the disease.

Notes

1   Access to a complete collection of print news media clippings was provided to the author by the AIDS Council of New South Wales for this period of AIDS reporting.

Chapter 5

AIDS Reporting in 1990

By the beginning of 1990, AIDS had almost completed its first decade of existence as a documented disease. Following the 'Grim Reaper' campaign, the Australian government continued to sponsor health education campaigns directed at the general public, while non-government organizations had been prominent in addressing gay men, male and female sex workers and injecting drug users with ongoing education programmes and support from the early years of the epidemic. The core message of the health education campaigns conducted by both government and non-government agencies in Australia was (and remains) the central warning that all sexually active individuals should be aware of AIDS, and should use condoms for all episodes of penetrative sex. A White Paper articulating the National HIV/AIDS Strategy was presented by the then Federal Health Minister, Neal Blewett, in August 1989. It rejected the imposition of a tight medical control over AIDS, and reinforced the principles of preventing HIV transmission through education and behavioural change and each individual's acceptance of responsibility for preventing infection. Between 1988 and 1990 five major AIDS education campaigns were sponsored by the Commonwealth government to warn of the risks involved in occasional injecting drug use and to reinforce the notion that non-drug-using heterosexuals could also be at risk if they practiced unsafe sex with partners who had shared injected needles and syringes. One advertizement showed an impassioned heterosexual couple falling onto a double bed studded with hundreds of hidden needles pointing threateningly upwards. Others featured testimonials, where heterosexuals who had contracted HIV told the story of how they came to be infected, or employed the 'vox pop' technique of interviewing people in the street about their attitudes to condoms.

By the early 1990s it appeared that existing programmes for

education, blood screening and needle-exchange had contained much of the spread of HIV in Australia. The annual incidence of AIDS rose sharply until 1988, but has levelled since then, suggesting a reduction in the rate of HIV transmission in the early or mid 1980s. While cases of AIDS due to heterosexual transmission and injecting drug use had slowly risen, they remained at a low level (Kaldor, McDonald, Blumer *et al.*, 1993). Gay men continued to comprise the vast majority of AIDS cases; by the end of December 1992 in Australia there were only 120 cases of AIDS attributed to heterosexual transmission alone, representing three per cent of all AIDS cases in Australia (National Centre in HIV Epidemiology and Clinical Research, 1993).

News coverage of AIDS in 1990

To compare more recent coverage of AIDS issues in the Australian press with that during the 'Grim Reaper' period, a seven-month period, March to September 1990 was analysed.[1] The most apparent difference is the diminishing in intensity of press interest in AIDS itself as a newsworthy item. A total of 2795 articles about AIDS were published during the seven months between March and September 1990 – far fewer articles than were published during the same period three years previously (Figure 5.1). It is clear from this same figure that although press attention to the syndrome rose steadily during the early years of AIDS reporting, it seemed to have peaked during the 'Grim Reaper' period, and by 1990 was in decline. For example, in April 1987, at the height of press attention to AIDS during the 'Grim Reaper' period of AIDS reporting, 940 AIDS items were published. The most AIDS items published in any one month during the later period of AIDS reporting was in August 1990, when almost half as many items (548) were published.

Press attention to AIDS as defined in quantitative terms is not the only important factor influencing public AIDS discourse. The types of topics and news actors receiving press attention, as well as the use of language to frame these topics are factors of equal importance in the construction of AIDS as a social phenomenon. As shown by the list of major topics receiving press attention in 1990 (Appendix 3), this later period differed somewhat from the early and middle years of AIDS as news in terms of the types of the issues and events reported. It is apparent by 1990 that the 'Gay Plague' metaphor had well and truly lost its currency in press accounts. This change in focus may be due in part to the intensity of news media coverage of the 'Grim Reaper'

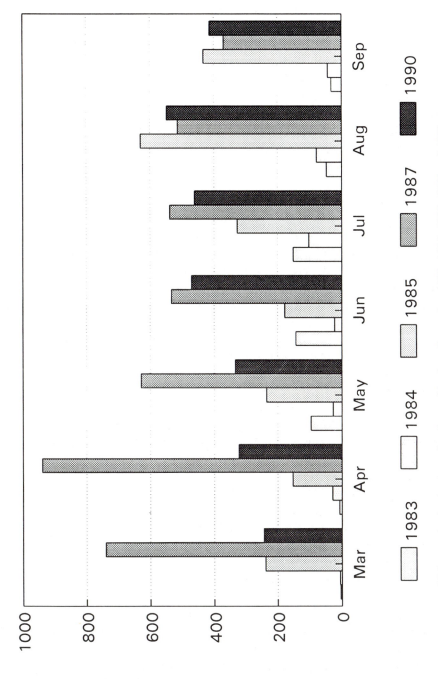

Figure 5.1   AIDS reporting in the Australian Press, March to September 1983, 1984, 1985, 1987 and 1990

campaign three years previously, which eclipsed the press' previous obsession with the theme of gay men and AIDS. However by 1990 the previously dominant theme – the threat posed by AIDS to heterosexuals – had also lost its newsworthiness. Articles dealing with HIV infection amongst gay men, injecting drug users and prostitutes, risk groups which had historically been the focus of news articles, were also few in number.

Adults with AIDS

As the list of major topics in Appendix 3 demonstrates, many news articles were about adults living with AIDS or infected with HIV. Most of these articles were general, dealing with such issues as the health problems of people living with AIDS, discrimination issues, decency campaigns against people living with AIDS who were gay men or injecting drug users, people living with AIDS lobby groups or support for people living with AIDS. The main focus of discourses on AIDS in the Australian press had thus moved from those *potentially* at risk of HIV infection back to those *already* infected. As the headlines reproduced below demonstrate, the emotive and overtly-judgemental rhetoric of the early period of AIDS reporting was much less in evidence when press accounts dealt with gay people living with AIDS. It is notable though that despite the insistence of many people with HIV infection or AIDS that they not be called 'victims' of AIDS, as this word implies passivity and domination by the virus, newspapers continued to use this terminology. People grouped under the generic titles of 'AIDS ill', 'AIDS carrier', 'AIDS sufferer' or 'AIDS victims' were largely portrayed sympathetically, or in a neutral fashion, as in the following headlines:

HOSPITAL 'TURNS GAY MAN WITH AIDS AWAY'

Sunday Times, 11 March 1990

AIDS ILL CRY OUT FOR HELP

Daily Sun, 27 March 1990

GAYS LEAD AIDS FIGHT

Daily Sun, 29 March 1990

VIGIL HONOURS MEMORY OF AIDS VICTIMS

Age, 21 May 1990

VICTIMS TELL TRAGIC STORIES

West Australian, 5 June 1990

DISCRIMINATION STILL ONE OF THE SIDE-EFFECTS OF AIDS

West Australian, 7 July 1990.

Personalization was used in several articles about gay people living with AIDS, in which the men were presented almost as martyrs, certain of death but spending their last days helping others, as in the following examples:

FRANCIS DEVOTES TIME LEFT TO EDUCATING OTHERS

Francis was 19 when he had his first HIV test, and the result was positive. He thought then that he had between six and 12 months to live ... His teenage problems with alcohol and drugs became steadily worse, and the next few years saw periods of homelessness and despair. Even the gay community in which he had mixed since his mid-teens, he said, was often too fearful to offer him support ... He wants to use what time he has left fighting discrimination and helping young people arm themselves with the education they need to avoid infection.

Sydney Morning Herald, 7 July 1990

ALIVE, BUT IN DEATH'S SHADOW

Robert Jarmen knows what it's like to have to take just one day at a time. He is one of about 40 people in Tasmania who have tested HIV positive. A member of the organization, People Living With AIDS Tasmania, 32-year-old Robert's world was shattered two years ago when he received the positive HIV results. Robert is gay and says he caught HIV/AIDS through high-risk sexual behaviour. Nowadays he still finds it difficult to accept. One of the concepts he finds hardest to deal with is the uncertainty surrounding his future. Despite working with the Tasmanian AIDS Council and facing HIV – AIDS issues every day, he says there are days when he wakes up and 'quite irrationally' denies it all for a couple of hours telling himself there is no such thing as HIV/AIDS ...

Hobart Mercury, 29 June 1990

SPREADING THE WORD ... AND THE QUILT

Eight years ago, Tony Bubner was diagnosed as being HIV positive ... He was sacked six months ago because two workmates were worried about infection. That, combined with losing the support of some people, left him depressed and ill. Mr Bubner, a homosexual, contracted the disease though sexual contact ... He is pale and has dark rings under his eyes – but despite this suffering and obvious emotional anguish, he aims to educate the community about AIDS ... Mr Bubner speaks to various Hobart business, health groups and youth groups about AIDS, and in particular, prevention. 'It is not a gay problem, it is one which the entire community has to address,' he said. ...

Hobart Mercury, 22 May 1990

All these stories demonstrate evidence of a certain sympathy towards the plight of gay men with HIV or AIDS, but there is also distance placed between the person living with AIDS and the readership. As argued in previous chapters, throughout the history of AIDS, the placing of responsibility for illness upon the individual has been a common discourse in government policy, AIDS education campaigns, and press accounts of AIDS. In the news stories excerpted above, even though the men were portrayed sympathetically, the mode of HIV transmission was made clear, implying their guilt for their illness: for example, 'Mr Bubner, a homosexual, contracted the disease through sexual contact Robert is gay and says he caught HIV/AIDS through high risk sexual behaviour'. There is no obvious need to state how people living with AIDS acquired HIV infection, but the drawing of distinctions between gay people living with AIDS and others, infected with HIV through alternative routes, was a commonplace feature of personalized stories. The original lexicon of AIDS, the previously dominant metaphors and phrases used to position discourses on AIDS in the early and 'Grim Reaper' periods of reporting, the common depiction of the retributive nature of the disease as a punishment for sexual sins, first homosexual, and in later years, heterosexual, ensured that these men could not easily be viewed as 'innocent victims'. There is, in these later accounts, the implicit assumption that gay people living with AIDS were being redeemed for their sins only through their efforts to help others.

It is worthy of note that the language employed in one of the articles serves both to reinforce the notion that AIDS is a gay men's disease, by its emphasis upon the way cited above in which 'AIDS sufferer Tony Bubner' contracted HIV, and denies that AIDS is limited to gay men by quoting Tony Bubner's assertions that, 'It is not a gay problem, it is one which the entire community has to address'. In its emphasis on Bubner's losing his job because 'two workmates were worried about infection', the spectre of casual transmission is raised but not countered. The article thus contains contradictory and confusing definitions of AIDS risk via casual transmission.

In contrast, those people living with AIDS who were infected through receiving contaminated blood products were presented in news accounts as 'innocent victims' and deserving not of punishment nor needful of redemption but rather compensation from the state for their illness. As noted by Juhasz (1990: 38), '[o]ther than babies who are cuter, and haemophiliacs who are already cursed with an unfortunate disease, blood transfusion recipients are the most holy of [people living with AIDS] . . . because their behaviour and lifestyle is unconnected to the contraction of the disease'. Press accounts emphasized that these people living with AIDS were not at fault for their illness because they had no control over the circumstances by which they became infected – they did not after all acquire HIV from 'high-risk sexual activities'. Several articles during 1990 described the attempts of such individuals to sue government authorities, blood banks or hospitals for negligence in providing them with infected blood products. In April 1990, for example, it was reported that more than

100 Australian people living with AIDS who contracted HIV through infected blood products had sued the Red Cross Blood Bank and Commonwealth Serum Laboratories for negligence. In June 1990, a 5-year-old boy in the USA was awarded $37.47 million after suing a hospital because they had supplied him with HIV-infected blood products from which he had developed AIDS, and in August an Australian married man with haemophilia sued the Red Cross for the same reason.

Reporting of these events was often quite factual and unemotive: items tended to provide the details of cases without the use of colourful rhetoric. Many headlines, however, contained language which implied that the newspapers in general supported the people living with AIDS' claims:

DYING GIRL AMONG 30 IN AIDS CLAIMS

Sydney Morning Herald, 29 March 1990

AIDS VICTIMS WIN ONE

Sydney Morning Herald, 6 April 1990

AIDS MAN SUES OVER 'BAD BLOOD'

Sun News-Pictorial, 14 July 1990

HAEMOPHILIAC CLAIMS BLOOD GAVE HIM AIDS VIRUS

Age, 16 August 1990.

The emphasis in these headlines upon AIDS 'victims' and 'dying' implies support and sympathy for people living with AIDS rather than the institutions they are suing, while the use of the terms 'haemophiliac' and 'bad blood' and the phrase 'blood gave him AIDS virus' clearly denotes that the people living with AIDS did not acquire HIV from sexual activities or injecting drug use (and by corollary, were not to blame for their illness, as were gay men, injecting drug users or promiscuous heterosexuals). For these particular people living with AIDS, the fault was purely external and therefore their condition could be blamed on someone or something else which 'gave' them the virus. Some articles were explicit on this point:

AIDS-CONTAMINATED BLOOD NOT ACT OF GOD, SAYS VICTIMS' MUM

The mother of two boys dying from the AIDS virus yesterday attacked moves by governments to guard against lawsuits from AIDS-infected haemophiliacs. [She] said the governments were denying their responsibility by the move. She said someone must be answerable to people who were innocently infected with AIDS ... 'My boys are dying a slow, painful death and someone is responsible, but nobody will admit to it. They had no choice – they were given infected blood products supposedly to save their lives. Maybe AIDS is an accident if an adult – a gay person or a druggie – knowingly takes a risk, but with haemophiliacs it can't be called an accident...'.

Courier-Mail, 12 June 1990

The use of accusative statements of blame and phrases such as 'not act of God . . . denying responsibility . . . someone must be answerable . . . innocently infected . . . someone is responsible . . . they had no choice . . . with haemophiliacs it can't be called an accident' denote an attempt to blame external forces, and to emphasize the essential innocence of HIV-infected people with haemophilia. To assert that these people living with AIDS 'had no choice' was to imply that other people living with AIDS (a 'gay person or a druggie') *did* have a choice, and that therefore, those people could not possibly blame others for their misfortune but must shoulder the blame for their illness themselves. This rhetoric is characterized by the need to explain the external cause of the boys' infection: it is an attempt to emphasize that this case is not one of individual culpability, but the fault of others.

The Sixth International Conference on AIDS, held in San Francisco in June 1990, occasioned attention from the press not only because of new data presented, but also because of controversy over the restrictive laws of the USA concerning travel of people with HIV infection and the vocal demonstrations staged by newly prominent gay activist and lobby groups such as ACT UP (AIDS Coalition to Unleash Power). When the meeting began, members of ACT UP staged protests effectively disrupting conference proceedings. The Fourth Australian National Conference on AIDS, held in Canberra in August, was also the scene of dramatic protests by the Australian chapter of ACT UP, which took over the opening ceremony of the conference.

Reporting of such protests varied between the sympathetic or neutral depiction of ill individuals with a just cause to the suggestion that AIDS protesters were needlessly militant and disruptive, noisy, bizarre, deviant, uncontrolled and wild, capable of 'sabotage' and posing a threat to the respectable institution of the medical conference, such as in the headlines

MILITANTS SABOTAGE AIDS CONFERENCE

Advertiser, 26 June 1990

and

ACTIVISTS THREATEN CONFERENCE ON AIDS

Canberra Times, 21 June 1990.

One newspaper account, published in the *Age* (21 June 1990) was headlined

WILD SCENE AT AIDS CONFERENCE HOTEL

and displayed a large photograph of a protester being dragged away by two burly policeman, their holstered guns clearly visible. The caption read, 'New York tussle: ACT UP members battle police during a protest against US immigration laws banning carriers of the AIDS virus'. The combination of headline, photograph and main text of this account represented gay protesters as uncivilized, uncontrollable, barbarian and deviant. The person shown being dragged away by the policemen looks violent, unconventional and somewhat androgynous. The police are very much in control of the situation, standing over the protester and grasping one arm each. The adjectives and phrases used in the headline and main text: 'ragged ... wild scene ... ear-splitting ... banging ... shrieking pandemonium ... smoke bomb ... wild looking ... pounded on drums ... chanted slogans ... violent confrontation'; the description of the protesters as blurring the boundaries of accepted gender roles and sexual behaviour: 'a hirsute male wearing a skirt and Panama hat, with "Tom" tattooed on the arm thumping a bass drum ... Hotel guests stared pop-eyed as two leather-clad women engaged in a long, passionate kiss under ACT UP's red and yellow banner', the description of people living with AIDS as 'carriers of the AIDS virus' all position the protesters as the alien and less than human 'other'. It is likely that such descriptions in the popular press undermined other accounts of gay people living with AIDS that were sympathetic and sought to normalize these individuals, serving to add to stereotypes of deviance and negative perceptions of gay activism as extremist and violent.

The propensity of the press to couch political dissent and protests in terms of conflict is a common stylistic feature of reporting. The effect of such portrayals upon the audience may well have been to suggest that progress in the fight against the epidemic was being hampered by petty politics, personality clashes and unacceptably extreme behaviour on the part of 'uncontrollable' gay activists. Such contentions of infighting and battles trivialize the issue, drawing audiences' attention away from more important aspects of the AIDS epidemic, such as the provision of funds for AIDS-related care.

Children with AIDS

In 1990, topics concerning the cases of individual children with AIDS received more press attention than those dealing with the individual cases of gay men living with AIDS. Significantly, the tone of articles about these children was far more sympathetic than those describing the plight of other people living with AIDS (especially gay men), and displayed a strong propensity towards reinforcing distinctions between the 'innocent' and the 'guilty' person, as, for example, in the headlines

MOTHER WATCHES SONS DIE – INNOCENT AIDS VICTIMS
Courier-Mail, 11 June 1990

and

TOO LITTLE TOO LATE: TRAGIC PLIGHT OF THE KIDS DOOMED TO AN AWFUL DEATH
Sunday Mail, 1 April 1990.

In April 1990, the death of Ryan White, an American adolescent with haemophilia who had contracted HIV through infected blood products and who had subsequently been subjected to discrimination from some residents of the small town in which he lived, received laudatory coverage:

US MOURNS YOUNG AIDS HERO
America's best-known teenage AIDS victim, Ryan White, died today after a six-year battle with the disease . . . White was given only 18 months to live once diagnosed, but outlived that deadline with an optimism and determination that impressed supporters worldwide.
Herald, 9 April 1990

BUSH PAYS TRIBUTE TO AIDS BATTLER
Ryan White, 18, the 'boy next door', who waged a highly publicized five-year battle against AIDS and the unreasoning fear of its victims, died yesterday. US President George Bush, who planted a tree in White's honour in Indianapolis last week, issued a brief statement saying his death 'reaffirms that we, as a people, must pledge to continue the fight against this dreaded disease'.
Daily Telegraph, 10 April 1990

TEENAGE AIDS HERO DIES
Sydney Morning Herald, 10 April 1990
A NATION WEEPS AS AIDS CLAIMS RYAN
Australian, 10 April 1990
TEENAGE MARTYR LOSES AIDS FIGHT
Courier-Mail, 10 April 1990
STARS SHONE BRIGHTLY THE DAY PLUCKY RYAN WAS BURIED: BOY WHO TAUGHT ENEMIES NOT TO FEAR AIDS
Sunday Times, 22 April 1990.

White, the 'boy next door', was portrayed as courageous, a martyr, a hero and a warrior who had lost the 'battle' he had waged against death. His fame was such that the American President paid 'tribute' to him, and 'a nation weeps' when he died. Apart from the young mother Suzi Lovegrove who died in 1987 and who was the subject of a moving television documentary (the press response to which was described in the previous chapter), no other person with AIDS to this point had received such praise and expressions of tragedy and sorrow in the Australian press as White in any of the reporting periods analysed.

Later that year, however, the tragic proportions of reportage of White's death was surpassed by the case of an Australian child. The last days of illness and the death of a 7-year-old Sydney girl Holly Johnson in August and September 1990 received enormous press attention. Holly's mother had died from AIDS after receiving infected blood products, and Holly contracted HIV from her mother's milk as an infant. She first received press attention in August when her case, suing a Sydney hospital for negligence, was lost. When her father sought publicity from the press in order to condemn publicly the court's decision, the child was thrust into the limelight. Holly Johnson's case was even more newsworthy for the Australian press than that of Ryan White's because she was Australian, much younger, and blonde and pretty before illness struck. Many articles about Holly were illustrated with photos of the tiny and extremely ill child accompanied by her grieving and despairing father; a widely syndicated photograph showed a frail Holly cowering sadly behind a blanket days before her death. Few readers could have failed to have been touched by the plight of the little girl.

Several press accounts following her death contrasted photographs of Holly before her illness, plump-cheeked and smiling, with the skeletal, huge-eyed figure she became as she neared death. Like accounts of White's death, the press dwelt in a sentimental manner upon Holly's courage, youth and innocence, and the tragedy of her death:

MY HEART ACHES FOR LITTLE HOLLY
Sunday Telegraph, 26 August 1990

LITTLE HOLLY DIES OF AIDS IN DAD'S ARMS
Courier-Mail, 4 September 1990

THE LAST GOODBYE: SHE LIFTED HER HAND TO GIVE A LITTLE WAVE
Daily Telegraph, 4 September 1990

EMOTIONAL FAREWELL TO BRAVE HOLLY: 'SHE REACHED OUT AND TOUCHED US ALL IN SOME WAY'
Daily Telegraph, 6 September 1990

'AN INNOCENT VICTIM' FAREWELLED
Sydney Morning Herald, 6 September 1990.

The newsworthiness of Holly's death was such that although few editorials dealing with AIDS appeared in 1990, several editorials published in tabloid newspapers were devoted to Holly's case. Two of these are reproduced below:

Editorial: HOLLY'S LEGACY

Brave seven-year-old Holly Johnson lost her short, sad fight against AIDS. She died peacefully in her sleep last night, surrounded by her family at her home in Wentworthville in Sydney's western suburbs. Holly contracted the disease from her mother Dannalee, who died 18 months ago after receiving a blood transfusion contaminated with AIDS. Her death is an enormous tragedy and a calamitous loss to her family and friends. Her legacy to the rest of us is an example of guts and determination – and a distressing reminder of the fact that the AIDS virus is a deadly and indiscriminate killer.

Daily Mirror, 4 September 1990

Editorial: HOLLY'S LEGACY

Little Holly Johnson's life was tragically brief. But she did not live – or die – in vain. Through her brave fight for life, she showed the world the human side of AIDS, and how the innocent can suffer. The community response to her plight showed the depths of caring in an often uncaring society and, thanks to Holly, many people now have a better understanding of AIDS. It is no longer seen as a sleazy virus that afflicts just drug addicts and homosexuals. It is seen for what it is: a living tragedy that condemns so many to a lingering death. Through Holly, many people have learned that AIDS victims deserve sympathy and dignity, not condemnation or callous disregard.

Daily Telegraph, 4 September 1990

Given that editorials offer the 'official' voice of the newspaper, seeking overtly to express an opinion, sum up the issues, or make a moral judgement or decision upon the issue, the stance chosen by those reproduced above is telling. Both editorials dwelt upon Holly's courage, youth and innocence, and the tragedy of her death. The use of the words and phrases 'brave', 'guts and determination', and 'fight' attest to Holly's courage. Her death was not only 'sad', but an 'enormous tragedy' and a 'calamitous loss' which was a 'distressing reminder' of the 'living tragedy of AIDS'.

Interestingly, both editorials emphasized the 'lessons' of Holly's death, and both were headlined 'HOLLY'S LEGACY'. Her death was said to demonstrate that AIDS can affect anyone (it is a 'deadly and indiscriminate killer'), that people living with AIDS 'deserve sympathy and dignity', that AIDS has a 'human side', that 'the innocent can suffer', and that AIDS is no longer 'seen as a sleazy virus'. It took the death of a blonde and pretty Australian child to emphasize these aspects: the death of yet another gay man or injecting drug user or even a 'promiscuous' heterosexual would not have sufficed. Indeed the deaths of many hundreds of Australian gay men from AIDS since the disease first appeared in Australia in 1982 may have received attention in terms of number of articles appearing in the press, but have never occasioned the same rhetoric of sentimentalism and tragedy.[2]

The absence of equivalent public distress and sympathy for others directly affected by AIDS, especially gay men, and the implications in press accounts of such individuals' moral turpitude and punishment for their deviant behaviour is evidence of whom the press, and by extension, society, considers important. For example, the second editorial above, in particular, is pejorative in its depiction of other people living with AIDS, who, it is implied, deserve their fate because of their 'sleazy' behaviour. Eight years after the first case of AIDS in Australia, these accounts contended that it was only when 'innocent' children were dying of AIDS, that society should be aware of the distress, privations and pain involved, and should extend its sympathy and help to such people. The implication is that if AIDS did affect 'just drug addicts and homosexuals' it would not be worthy of comment.

AIDS as a weapon

Two newly dominant metaphors to emerge during the later period of AIDS reporting were 'AIDS as weapon' and 'AIDS as crime', stemming from a number of attempts by individuals to perpetrate crimes using as weapons needles allegedly filled with HIV-infected blood. In July 1990, three robberies in Sydney using syringes attracted press attention, and newspaper articles also reported the story of a Melbourne store-owner who was held up by a thief with a syringe he claimed to be infected with HIV. As a consequence of publicity around this Melbourne case, the Victorian and New South Wales state governments undertook to review their murder laws to cover such actions. In August and September there were several more hold-ups featuring syringes, followed by press calls for a legal response formally acknowledging syringes used in such a way as weapons. The language used in press accounts dwelt upon the new meaning of syringes as lethal weapons:

SYRINGE 'A SHOTGUN'

Sun News-Pictorial, 20 June 1990

BLOOD-FILLED SYRINGES IN CRIME WAR

Daily Mirror, 30 July 1990

SYRINGE ATTACKS TO BE MURDER

Launceston Examiner, 31 July 1990

NEEDLES DEADLIER THAN GUN

Daily Telegraph, 31 July 1990

NEEDLE BANDITS 'LETHAL'

Sun News-Pictorial, 1 August 1990

SYRINGE BANDITS STRIKE

Sunday Territorian, 19 August 1990.

It may be contended that this new conception of danger served to add to the stigmatizing of AIDS, adding to the imagery of crime, deviance, terror and general societal lack of control surrounding the disease. One article was particularly explicit in utilizing these metaphors: 'Police can shoot a criminal using a syringe as a weapon if it is a threat to the public, the NSW Police Association has said. "It is the same as if the person was carrying a double-barrelled shot-gun", association deputy president Phil Holder said yesterday' (*Sun News-Pictorial*, 20 June 1990).

In May 1990, the issue of AIDS as a weapon in prisons was given further impetus when an HIV-infected prisoner was convicted in the USA of trying to murder a jail guard by biting him. That month, the New South Wales Minister for Corrective Services announced that all prisoners in the state would be required to undergo HIV antibody testing but would not be issued with condoms. In July 1990, a Sydney prison officer, Geoffrey Pearce, was allegedly stabbed in the buttocks by a prisoner wielding an HIV-infected syringe. This event received a large amount of press coverage, with headlines focusing upon the 'horror' and 'terror' experienced by Pearce when waiting for the HIV antibody test results:

GUARD FACES 3 MONTHS OF HELL AFTER AIDS JAB

Australian, 24 July 1990

THREE MONTHS OF HELL FOR GEOFF: AIDS ATTACK PRISON OFFICER'S FEARS

Daily Mirror, 24 July 1990

AGONIZING WAIT FOR RESULT OF LIFE-OR-DEATH TESTS: AIDS-JAB WARDER TELLS OF TERROR

Daily Telegraph, 24 July 1990.

Reports of the attack were followed later that month by coverage of a strike by New South Wales prison warders, who called for the segregation of HIV-infected prisoners to protect their safety. In September the positive result of Pearce's HIV antibody test was released, and all metropolitan newspapers featured large articles about the case, with accompanying photographs of Pearce looking introspective. Headlines were sympathetic, emphasizing his courage, the 'agony' he was experiencing in dealing with the diagnosis of HIV seropositivity, and his status as an 'innocent' victim of HIV infection.

JAB VICTIM HAS AIDS VIRUS: SYRINGE NOW A FEARED WEAPON
West Australian, 1 September 1990
AIDS AGONY: JABBED WARDER TESTS POSITIVE
Daily Telegraph, 1 September 1990
BRAVE YOUNG WARDER FACES UP TO HIV
Australian, 2 September 1990.

It is notable that in several of these articles Pearce was quoted as stressing that 'Just because I am HIV-positive doesn't mean I am going to die' and 'I've got a very long life ahead of me'. These positive assertions counter the vast body of negative statements typical of press accounts of AIDS that the disease is an inevitable death sentence (especially when used in the context of gay men and children with HIV infection). The conception of AIDS as a manageable, if chronic and debilitating condition had been relatively uncommon in press accounts up to this point. It was perhaps emphasized in press accounts in Pearce's case in order to demonstrate his masculine courage, bravery and lack of passivity in the face of his predicament.

Following the announcement of Pearce's seropositivity there was extended debate in the press concerning the control of infected prisoners and mooted penalties for assault with infected blood. It was revealed in press reports that more prison officers had been tested for HIV after being assaulted by prisoners with syringes, and that a number of officers in New South Wales prisons had resigned because of fear of infection. Headlines emphasized the fears now faced by prison workers:

JAIL OFFICERS NEED AIDS PROTECTION
Herald, 7 September 1990
AIDS ALERT: FEAR GRIPS JAILS OVER 'JAB' WARDER
Sun News-Pictorial, 1 September 1990
WARDER QUITS AFTER SYRINGE STAB
Daily Mirror, 17 September 1990.

Prisoners themselves were portrayed in many press accounts as violent desperados and drug addicts, worthy of little sympathy even if HIV-infected, while prison workers were portrayed as heroes, fighting to maintain law and order amongst their unruly charges, and fearing for their lives while performing such duties. These themes were particularly dominant in an editorial concerning the issue excerpted below:

JAIL OFFICERS NEED AIDS PROTECTION
The dreadful menace of AIDS looms large in everyday Australian life. Make no mistake: not only those who ignore official advice on how to avoid the fatal disease have been at risk. This week the nation mourned the loss of a little girl, Holly Johnson, who

as a baby caught the disease at the breast of her mother, who, in turn, caught AIDS from a blood transfusion. Last week Australians learned a 21-year-old NSW prison officer, Geoffrey Pearce, has the killer disease after a prisoner stabbed him with a blood-filled syringe . . . Many prisoners are drug addicts who share needles which they conceal. Apart from deliberate attacks by prisoners, warders sometimes stick themselves accidentally while searching cells or clothing, then spend an agonizing wait until tests show if they are infected. A total of six NSW prison officers have been jabbed. In Pentridge an infected prisoner worked in the officers' canteen for weeks, before a test to which he had consented revealed he had AIDS. Understandably, prison officers want regular compulsory testing of all prisoners. But thanks largely to the misguided efforts of civil libertarians and gay activists, who have clouded so much of the AIDS priorities which places the public interest last, compulsory testing has been rejected. But what about the individual rights of people, such as prison officers and medical staff, exposed by their jobs to the unacceptable risk of the unknown? Surely they have a right to protection?

Herald, 7 September 1990

The editorial is overtly extremely sympathetic to the cause of prison officers. The headline of the editorial – 'JAIL OFFICERS NEED AIDS PROTECTION' – unequivocally states the intention to put the case of the officers over that of the prisoners. The editorial is completely one-sided, representing officers as innocent bystanders 'with a right to protection', who are facing death 'at the end of a needle'. The prisoners are, by corollary, guilty and undeserving of any rights, including the right not to be compulsorily tested for HIV. The case of the infected prisoner who 'worked in the officers' canteen for weeks' before he was found to be HIV antibody positive is cited, raising the spectre of casual transmission – for how else did this prisoner pose a threat to the officers? The use of the term 'drug addicts' to describe the prisoners is pejorative, again implying that their lives are relatively unimportant compared to those of the more valued prison officers.

Pearce's innocent status as a person living with AIDS is underlined in the editorial by the direct comparison of his plight with that of the child Holly Johnson, already established by the press as the epitome of the innocent and brave victim of AIDS whose death was so tragic that 'a nation mourned [her] loss'. His exposure to HIV infection is held up as the example of the danger faced by all prison officers, serving to obfuscate the significant social and political aspects of the officer–prisoner relationship, and the reasons why prisoners may feel provoked into attacking officers with syringes. Compulsory testing is put forward as the solution to HIV amongst prisoners, with those who oppose such coercive measures denigrated and marginalized as 'civil libertarians and gay activists'. Injecting drug use among prisoners is presented as a problem affecting prison staff rather than prisoners themselves, while the need for needle exchange and provision of condoms is not recognized as an important issue in the debate.

It is also notable that although the editorial asserts that the 'dreadful menace of AIDS looms large in everyday life', the discussion largely focuses upon AIDS issues in prisons, institutions that are not a feature of most people's everyday experiences. The discourse of AIDS as a threat to all Australians, dominant in press accounts during the 'Grim Reaper' period of reporting, finds echoes in this editorial, as does the ideology of victim-blaming, which places responsibility upon individuals to heed government warnings and protect themselves from HIV infection: 'not only those who ignore official advice on how to avoid the fatal disease have been at risk'. AIDS risk is represented not only as a threat against which the individual should protect him or herself (the dominant theme of the 'Grim Reaper' era of reporting) and which is largely under control, but also as a lurking threat being incubated in the nation's prisons.

The global spread of AIDS

The holding of three major AIDS conferences (the Sixth International AIDS Conference, the Fourth Australian National AIDS Conference and the First Conference on AIDS in Asia and the Pacific) during 1990 resulted in a number of newspaper articles based on presentations given at these meetings. The major focus in many of these articles was the global spread of the epidemic. Such reports tended to suggest that the AIDS epidemic was less of a problem in Australia than previously predicted, while elsewhere in the world, especially in developing countries in Asia and Africa, the epidemic continued to worsen. The following headlines contributed to this representation of the out-of-control spread of AIDS elsewhere in the world:

WORLDWIDE AIDS EPIDEMIC 'OUT OF CONTROL'
Sunday Age, 18 March 1990
AFRICA'S GRIM REAPER: AIDS IS RUNNING RAMPANT
Sunday Mail, 22 April 1990
THIRD WORLD FACES 'ATOMIC BOMB' EFFECT OF AIDS
Advertiser, 25 June 1990
ASIA IS AIDS LATEST TARGET
Sun Herald, 29 July 1990
AIDS SURGES IN ASIA, AFRICA, SAYS WHO
Age, 2 August 1990
HIV EPIDEMIC SWEEPING ASIA
Sydney Morning Herald, 6 August 1990
CONCERN OVER RAPID RISE OF AIDS IN THE PACIFIC
Newcastle Herald, 6 August 1990.

These may be compared with contemporary and more reassuring headlines describing the state of the AIDS epidemic in Australia:

STUDY FINDS AIDS NUMBERS DOWN
Daily News, 4 May 1990
EXPECTED SPREAD OF DISEASE 'HAS NOT EVENTUATED'
Advertiser, 31 May 1990
AIDS SPREAD MAY HAVE LEVELLED OFF
Sydney Morning Herald, 31 May 1990
AUSSIE AIDS DIFFERENT, SAYS EXPERT
Hobart Mercury, 20 June 1990
WORLD AIDS TREND DEFIED IN AUSTRALIA
Daily Telegraph, 23 June 1990.

These latter articles went on to make reassuring statements:

> The spread of AIDS appeared to have plateaued in Australia and could be on the verge of a downturn, a senior Federal Government health official said yesterday. Commonwealth chief medical adviser Dr Tony Adams said the latest figures suggested earlier fears about the virus's impending rapid spread among drug users and the general community had not eventuated.
> *Advertiser*, 31 May 1990

> Australia is defying the predicted pattern of AIDS in the developed world, the Sixth International Conference on AIDS was told yesterday. While countries like the US have seen the virus spread among intravenous drug users and into the heterosexual population, the epidemic in Australia seems to have remained confined largely to homosexual men.
> *Daily Telegraph*, 23 June 1990

Compared with the panic statements made about the spread of AIDS throughout Australian society in the 'Grim Reaper' period, such contentions are striking for their newfound complacency and lack of alarm. As described in Chapter Four under the shadow of the 'Grim Reaper' AIDS was said to be 'out of control ... here to stay ... a potential holocaust' from which 'we are all in danger'. By 1990, press accounts inferred that Australia had emerged victorious from the epidemic which had been 'defied ... not eventuated ... levelled off ... plateaued ... on the verge of a downturn ... remained confined'. Just as direct quotes from 'AIDS experts' were used to fuel panic statements about apocalyptic visions during the 'Grim Reaper' period, and quantification rhetoric was commonly used to emphasize the threat posed by AIDS to all Australians, so similar persuasive devices were employed in 1990 to reassure the Australian population that the threat of exponential spread of HIV in Australia seemed unlikely. As when AIDS was first discovered and the first accounts of the new disease appeared in the press, the epidemic, it was suggested in these more recent accounts, had once again become the disease of the 'other': that is, a problem in far-off other countries but not at home, and an issue 'confined largely to homosexual men' but posing little threat to the 'general population'.

It could be argued that press insistence in such accounts that AIDS was a far greater problem in developing countries than in Australia had good factual basis. Global estimates of the spread of infection worldwide at that time indicated that Oceania was the least affected region in the world, and that in comparison to sub-Saharan Africa, the AIDS epidemic in Australia was of little magnitude, both in terms of absolute numbers and *per capita* (Chin, 1990). However, it is telling that as Appendix 3 demonstrates, most topics in items about AIDS printed in the Australian press were concerned with events or people in Australia, the USA and other western countries. Despite the enormity of the problems posed by AIDS in sub-Saharan African countries and the growing threat of devastation in South-East Asia, comparatively few articles were devoted to this dimension of the epidemic. The tragedy of the illness of a small number of western children with AIDS was greatly emphasized over that of the thousands of gay men and African men, women and children dying of the disease.

AIDS education campaigns

Government-sponsored AIDS education campaigns continued to receive press attention, especially if they were perceived as controversial. No campaigns run during the 1990 study period, however, were the subject to the same degree of publicity accorded the 1987 'Grim Reaper' campaign. Press accounts were also less supportive and more critical of government-sponsored campaigns in 1990 compared with their whole-hearted support of the 'Grim Reaper' campaign. Press reports of public health AIDS education campaigns tended either to describe them factually and report that a new campaign had been released, or to report upon controversy caused by campaigns considered too *outre* for public consumption. One such controversial campaign, causing several letters both of complaint and of support to newspapers, was the Commonwealth Department of Community Services and Health's nationwide campaign released in June 1990. This included television advertizements which showed 'real' people with HIV recounting how they had been infected, and a series of humorous 'vox pop' about attitudes to condoms. One of the most prominent people to complain about these advertizements was the National President of the Australian Medical Association, who asserted that the campaign would cause worry but not control the disease. Clergymen from the Catholic Church criticized the campaign for promoting sexual irresponsibility and condom use as the only answer to AIDS, rather than exploring the alternatives of chastity and monogamy.

Some of the criticism directed at the Federal campaign was that more money should be spent on AIDS education campaigns directed at specific groups at greatest risk from infection, such as gay men and injecting drug users, rather than the general heterosexual population (again a change in sentiment compared with the 'Grim Reaper' period of AIDS reporting). Despite these criticisms, the health education campaigns that received the most controversy during 1990 were those aimed specifically at gay men and were produced by non-government AIDS support organizations. In August 1990, the opposition party in the state of Western Australia alleged that photographs used to illustrate gay-oriented safer sex booklets distributed by the Western Australian AIDS Council were too explicit, and during July and August there was reported controversy in Victoria about a poster directed at gay men produced by the Victorian AIDS Council which showed young men kissing. Headlines referred to the outrageous and controversial nature of the subject matter of these educational materials:

SAFE SEX ADS FURORE
Sunday Mail, 3 June 1990

ANTI-AIDS CONDOM ADS UNDER ATTACK
Sunday Mail, 3 June 1990

BISHOPS UPSET BY CONDOM ADS
Canberra Times, 6 June 1990

CHURCH ATTACKS AIDS ADS
Daily Mirror, 6 June 1990

KISSING MEN IN AIDS AD SPARKS PROTESTS
Advertiser, 26 July 1990

AIDS AD ROW: 'BLATANT' POSTER SLAMMED
Sun News-Pictorial, 26 July 1990

OUTRAGE OVER MALE KISS AND TELL AIDS AD
Australian, 26 July 1990

AIDS POSTER STARTS A ROW OVER SAFE-SEX CAMPAIGN
Age, 26 July 1990

AIDS ADS OVERSTEP THE MARK
Sunday Sun, 29 July 1990

'OBSCENE' AIDS BOOK ATTACKED
Northern Territory News, 6 August 1990.

Although the 'Gay Plague' metaphor is not overtly apparent here, there were still overt prurience and titillation in the language used: 'obscene . . . kissing men . . . male kiss and tell . . . blatant'. The desire to suggest conflict between Church and State and between gay organizations and the general population is also apparent in the use of the words, 'upset . . . furore . . . attacked . . . protests . . . outrage . . . row . . . slammed' in the headlines. Such negative coverage of education materials directed at the gay population rather than heterosexuals is further evidence of news media discrimination against homosexual sexuality, and their tendency to represent or treat such depictions as 'obscenity' or 'pornography' rather than as valid educational material; see also, Watney (1987: Chapter 4).

The valorization of medical science

Over the first decade of AIDS reporting, the advances made by scientists and medical researchers in searching for a cure for HIV infection or a vaccine to protect against infection, or treatments for AIDS-related conditions, gained press attention in varying degrees. In the 'Grim Reaper' period, the emphasis upon individual behavioural change and preventive health efforts dominated press accounts of AIDS, but 1990 was characterized by increasing reports about medical science's attempts to counteract the epidemic, and the efforts of AIDS activist groups to speed the approval of new drugs to treat HIV infection and AIDS symptoms. Many of these discoveries were made by British, French and American researchers, and several were reported in the context of conference proceedings when the results of latest studies were made public.

As shown in Appendix 3, the major topics of each month between March and August 1990 included several dealing with the progress of medical science in limiting the transmission of HIV or in treating AIDS-related conditions. In March 1990, it was reported that an AIDS vaccine developed by an Austrian drug company protected chimpanzees against HIV, in April French researchers succeeded in preventing HIV from reproducing in a human cell and in May the apparent success of the new drug DDI in treating HIV infection received press attention. In June, the International AIDS Conference was told that an American-developed vaccine which had been tested on mice could become widely available in two years. In July, a new British vaccine was reported to be tested soon on humans and articles reported that a compound extracted from a Queensland marine sponge might provide a cure for HIV infection. In August, the British vaccine again received press attention, as did the efforts of American researchers in developing a synthetic molecule that attaches to HIV and prevents it from spreading to other cells.

As in previous years, medical research was generally reported uncritically, with the use of rhetoric suggesting that new drugs or vaccines offered a solution, or 'hope' for the worldwide AIDS crisis. Researchers were presented as heroes, actively working against the clock to produce solutions, as the following headlines demonstrate:

GENETIC SCISSORS COULD KILL HEART OF AIDS VIRUS

Australian, 11 March 1990

US DEVELOPS GENE TO CUT AND DESTROY AIDS VIRUS

Age, 19 March 1990

SCIENCE PUTS AIDS ON HOLD

Sun, 9 April 1990

HOPES RISE IN BATTLE TO DEFEAT AIDS

Daily Sun, 10 April 1990

DRUG ADDS NEW HOPE IN AIDS VIRUS BATTLE

Advertiser, 11 May 1990

TESTS FIND A MARINE KILLER FOR THE AIDS VIRUS

Age, 19 July 1990

CSIRO [Commonwealth Scientific and Industrial Research Organisation] JOINS RACE TO FIND AIDS VACCINE

Australian, 16 August 1990.

Such imagery also informed reporting in the main texts:

NEW VACCINE BUILDS AIDS-FIGHTING CELLS

An experimental vaccine has helped healthy human volunteers to produce antibodies which seek out and destroy AIDS-infected cells . . . Killer T cells are the stronger type of protection because they are aimed at infected cells . . . [the vaccine] was shown to stimulate the immune system to kill infected cells.

Australian, 9 June 1990

The language used in the above headlines and excerpt draws upon the metaphor of 'medicine as war against disease' as witnessed in the use of active terms and noun phrases such as 'cut and destroy . . . AIDS virus battle . . . killer for the AIDS virus . . . AIDS-fighting cells . . . aimed at infection cells . . . stronger type of protection . . . kill the heart of AIDS virus . . . kill infected cells . . . battle to defeat AIDS'. Here, drugs are personified as moral crusaders, depicted in an active role in seeking out and destroying the forces of evil which are killing body cells but seem also passive and vulnerable to attack from the drugs. The drugs are thus presented as extensions of the more general medical and scientific 'know-how' that is benefiting society.

Several articles featured stereotypical icons of medical science, such as microscopes, test tubes, men (and very occasionally women) in white lab coats and computer images of blood cells or HIV itself. As well as employing these icons, such articles used highly technical jargon and acronyms, incomprehensible to the lay audience, to dazzle the reader with science:

> A senior research scientist with the CSIRO division of chemicals and polymers, Dr Sid Marcuccio, said the new anti-AIDS drugs were classified as HeteroPolyAnions and were believed to be a more effective variation from HPA-23, developed by the French ... The Melbourne University physicist who first applied SPM technology to anti-AIDS drugs in cells, Dr Marian Cholewa, said images of drugs inside a cell were produced by bombarding blood samples with nuclear particles called protons from a five million-volt accelerator attached to the SPM.
>
> *Australian*, 16 August 1990

In this particular article, scientists/researchers were portrayed as dynamic through the repeated use of active verbs; they are said to 'open [a] window to watch anti-virus drugs work inside blood cells', they have 'developed drugs' and joined the 'international race for an AIDS vaccine' by 'using technology'. Drugs were personalized as the assistants of the scientists/researchers 'working' to 'prevent HIV from replicating in human blood cell samples'. The routine employment of such rhetoric to valorize the efforts of 'Science' within the AIDS epidemic is worthy of comment. That science is so often presented unproblematically in the popular press, demonstrates contemporary society's obeisance towards technological medicine. Medical 'breakthroughs' are routinely reported in tones of awe and wonder, implying the scientists have taken on the role of saints in performing miracles and restoring life. The use of scientific jargon in articles, such as 'HeteroPolyAnions', 'HPA-23', 'SPM technology' and 'protons' in the above excerpt, shroud these deeds in mystery. It may be contended that throughout 1990 continuing valorization of science in AIDS discourses in the press served to detract the audience's attention away from the preventive issues to do with the syndrome, since such discourse implies that behaviour change is only a short-term necessity until science is able to provide a solution to AIDS. Rhetorics of 'hope' and 'war' combine together to suggest that it is only a matter of time before science will rise to the occasion.

AIDS in the health care setting

One of the main changes over time is the fluctuation in the intensity of press attention to different 'risk groups' in Australian AIDS reportage. The new issue of AIDS as a weapon, in concert with the representation of prison officers as a major new risk group for AIDS, was detailed earlier. Another issue which received greater attention in the press in 1990 concerned the dangers posed by HIV in the health care setting, both for health care workers and for their patients. Major topics included the case in March of a New York doctor who sued a hospital at which she had worked after she allegedly acquired HIV infection from a needle-stick injury. The case was settled out of court. In May, the Australian Medical Association (AMA) was reported as recommending the immediate administration of AZT to health workers with needle-stick injuries. In the same month, the President of this same Association attracted headlines when he called for a compulsory six-monthly HIV antibody test for all doctors and nurses working in risk areas, as well as for all patients undergoing surgery. In June, the press reported the first case of an Australian health worker contracting HIV through a needle-stick injury, and reports followed in July concerning the cases of eight Sydney doctors who had been infected in the same way. The AMA subsequently called again for routine tests of all patients before surgery.

The way in which the issue of health care workers and AIDS was represented was similar in many respects to the press reporting of prison workers and AIDS described earlier. Both groups were portrayed as bravely and nobly courting danger in the course of their duties, the patient in this case being the source of danger as evidenced by the following headlines:

DYING DOCTOR IN AIDS 'WIN': SECRET PAYOUT ENDS INFECTED NEEDLE CASE
Daily News, 9 March 1990

DOCTORS TO GET AIDS PROTECTION
Launceston Examiner, 29 June 1990

DOCTORS 'LIVE IN FEAR OF AIDS' AFTER NEEDLE JABS
Advertiser, 6 July 1990

AIDS THREAT HANGS OVER EIGHT DOCTORS
Daily Telegraph, 6 July 1990.

However, this noble depiction of health care workers was somewhat tarnished when the attitudes of general practitioners to HIV-infected patients were reported in a study published in the *Medical Journal of Australia* in July 1990. This study found that approximately a quarter of the general practitioners surveyed did not want to treat seropositive people for fear of becoming infected themselves. Headlines such as

STUDY EXPOSES GPS' WEAKNESS ON AIDS
Sydney Morning Herald, 2 July 1990

and

AIDS IGNORANCE AMONG GPS 'WIDESPREAD'
Advertiser, 2 July 1990

subsequently inferred that the practitioners should know better. The AMA's position was further undermined in July, when reports were published of an American woman who claimed to have contracted HIV from her dentist during a tooth extraction. Articles published in September subsequently alleged that two other patients of the same dentist had tested positive for HIV antibodies.

These reports served firstly to support the dominant ideology of health workers, especially physicians, as caring, high status individuals who were placed at risk of HIV infection by their patients, but could not themselves pose a risk by virtue of their lack of deviancy. It is interesting, however, that this dominant discourse was later challenged when cases were reported of patients contracting HIV infection from their dentist, and when general practitioners were shown to be discriminatory in their attitudes towards people living with AIDS. The unusualness of this situation: of doctors and other health professionals behaving in a socially unexpected manner and threatening the health of their patients, attracted press attention, and for a time such individuals were portrayed not as victims requiring 'protection', but as the perpetrators of infection and discrimination.

Summary

AIDS reporting in 1990 articulated a diverse and often contradictory range of discourses on AIDS, many of which served to distance the general readership from viewing the disease as relevant to themselves. AIDS reporting was characterized by a plurality of topics, most of which centred around the plight of those who had acquired HIV medically, the issue of AIDS in prisons, AIDS policy and politics, the spread of HIV in developing nations, the advances of drugs and medical science, the use of AIDS as a weapon and AIDS in the health care setting. Health education programmes as a means of preventing AIDS lost much of their primacy, while the progress of medical science in fighting AIDS and HIV infection was valorized.

By 1990 the apocalyptic visions of the future dominating in the 'Grim Reaper' period had disappeared, to be replaced by complacency and routinization, the notion that AIDS was 'someone else's problem'. Although a high level of press attention was paid to people living with AIDS, and their stories personalized, most of the individuals concerned were not portrayed in a way which would encourage general audiences to identify with them. AIDS had again become the disease of the 'other': the gay man coping with impending death, the person with haemophilia seeking compensation for HIV infection contracted through blood products, the gay activist; the prisoner and the prison officer; victims of violent crime; the population of Africa and South-East Asia. Even when the 'innocent child' archetype received press attention, it was emphasized that transmission had occurred via infected blood products, a route which no longer constitutes a source of infection in Australia.

The initial over-riding impression of a comparison of the 1990 articles with those published in 1986 to 1988 is the paucity of metaphors used. Articles published in 1990 were much more prosaic, with little use of metaphor compared with previous years of AIDS reporting. Instead of being used metaphorically, the word 'AIDS' was more commonly used as an adjective, as in the following phrases: 'AIDS victim . . . AIDS fear . . . AIDS girl . . . AIDS issue . . . AIDS appointment . . . AIDS drugs'. While a few common and established metaphors continued to be used, including 'AIDS is an enemy', 'AIDS is a killer' and 'AIDS is death', the panic-stricken visions of the epidemic changing society, and metaphors signifying danger to all, were rarely used. Two new metaphors to be established in the press in 1990, emerging from the spate of incidents in which blood-filled needles were used to threaten or attack, were 'AIDS as weapon' and 'AIDS as crime', serving once again to reinforce a marginalization and stigmatization of AIDS risk.

General conclusions: changes in AIDS reporting over the first decade

Weeks (1989) has identified three main periods of AIDS history in Britain and the USA between the years 1980 and 1988. The first period, from 1980 to 1982–3, he entitles the 'Dawning Crisis' period, in which AIDS emerged as a new and alarming epidemic. The second period, the 'Moral Panic' era, he places from the beginning of 1983 and the first isolation of identification of the virus believed to cause AIDS. The third period, post-1986, characterized by belated government response in the form of health education campaigns, he entitles 'Crisis Management'. This broad framework by which to order the history of AIDS is applicable to the way in which the disease was greeted in Australia. However, while the major thematic patterns of AIDS reporting appear to be common to the news media in Australia, Britain and the USA, there were major differences in the manner in which the Australian, American and British press reported AIDS which parallels differences in policy orientation.

In most respects, Australian policy was more progressive than that of Britain and the USA because of such factors as the benefit of forewarning, the greater liberalism of the Federal Labor government which held power in Australia from 1983 onwards, the inclusion of gay men into policy-making bodies, the tradition of state-provided health care and the lack of a strong political presence of radical religious conservatives (Altman, 1988). As noted in Chapter One, unlike the Australian press coverage of the 'Grim Reaper' campaign during 1987, British press coverage of AIDS education campaigns during 1988–90 was characterized by a plurality of interests and controversy. The emergence of a dominant New Right in the British political scene in the 1980s and its emphasis on issues to do with 'the family' and its enemies was not reflected in Australia. Australia did not possess a powerful political faction to dispute issues of heterosexual risk or to make homophobic statements publicly. The greater dichotomy between the liberal and the conservative press in Britain, which is not so evident in Australia, allowed the 'myth of heterosexual AIDS' issue to be split between two opposing camps and provide ongoing fuel for controversy and debate in the British news media (Murray, 1991; Beharrell, 1991; Berridge, 1991). In Australia loss of interest in the issue proved more damaging to the government's aims than did high levels of controversy, as press attention turned away from heterosexual sexual activity as a risk factor, towards the plight of children with AIDS and other issues.

In the USA the conservatism of the Reagan and Bush administrations in power during the 1980s, both of which were influenced by the Moral Majority lobby's aversion to the public discussion of homosexuality, resulted in AIDS issues being generally neglected and minimized to an even greater extent than in Australia (Altman, 1986). American government policy ranged from non-existent to punitive; for example, President Ronald Reagan's only public address on AIDS in 1987 called for mandatory testing for certain social groups such as prisoners and immigrants, and suggested routine testing for marriage license applicants (Adam, 1989: 11). American news media coverage of AIDS has correspondingly been characterized by conservative moralistic statements concerning male homosexual practices and the privileging of sexual abstinence as the preferred preventive strategy against HIV transmission (Albert, 1986a, 1986b; Baker, 1986; Nelkin, 1991). To counter the apathy of the American government and the silence of the news media, ACT UP was forced to create attention in the late 1980s by staging protests and media stunts to attract news coverage (Nelkin, 1991; Colby and Cook, 1991). While Australia has a chapter of ACT UP, it is much smaller and less active than the American group, perhaps because there has been less need for activists to challenge AIDS policy as there is much greater Australian government support for people living with AIDS and a higher level of media coverage of AIDS issues.

Recent cultural theory emphasizes that there is scope for admitting difference and contradiction in the ideologies and discourses reproduced in media texts. Many aspects of AIDS discourse in the news have exemplified evidence of contradictory ideologies and discourses at the site of news accounts of the disease, providing scope for different audiences to draw different meanings from the texts. In the Australian press' coverage of AIDS, the 'Gay Plague' metaphor had initially framed AIDS as news. This original social construction of AIDS meant that the 'Grim Reaper' period of AIDS reporting was marked by its insistence that AIDS was *not* a gay disease, but now was a disease affecting everyone. A major binary opposition was reversed: AIDS moved from being a disease of the 'other' to a disease of the 'self'. But even during this process, the original formulation of AIDS was never far from the surface, for reports constantly harkened back to the first lexical formulae developed to make sense of AIDS. The meanings of AIDS risk as represented in the Australian press during the periods of reporting examined were therefore contradictory, confusing and anxiety-provoking, promoting lack of adherence to a coherent theme, moving from positioning deviant outgroups as the only members of the population at risk from HIV infection, to an intense focus upon the threat posed to everybody, and back again to complacency.

The apocalyptic imagery of the 'Grim Reaper' period simply could not be sustained, especially since the numbers of heterosexuals falling ill or testing positive for HIV antibodies in the months and years following the campaign did not match the alarmist government warnings. Estimations of numbers of those who had HIV or AIDS in the Australian population, as reported by the press, veered wildly from one month to the next. Together with the pre-established discourses on sexuality, homosexuality, deviance, death and punishment which were hegemonic during the early years of AIDS reporting, personal experience (that is, not knowing anyone who was heterosexual and who had HIV or AIDS), interpersonal communication and people's natural desire to discount unpleasant possibilities, all may have served to compete against the predominant preferred theme of AIDS as a threat to all which emerged in 1987. In the face of such opposition, it is perhaps not surprising that the 'apocalyptic visions' theme was unable to be sustained for long, and that reporting of AIDS in 1990 reverted to representing those at risk from AIDS as the 'other'.

Notes

1 This period of reporting was chosen on the basis of collaboration with a colleague who had been funded by a Commonwealth AIDS Research Committee grant to conduct an analysis of Australian news coverage of AIDS. The funding provided for a clippings service to supply print news media AIDS items for seven months.
2 At the time when these news accounts were published, there were almost 2000 cases of AIDS identified in Australia, of which 88 per cent were gay or bisexual men. In comparison, there were only 17 cases of children with AIDS (National Centre in HIV Epidemiology and Clinical Research's Australian HIV Surveillance Report, Vol. 6, Supplement 1), 1990.

Chapter 6

AIDS, Textuality and Ideology

To understand the linguistic choices made in news reports of AIDS, it is important to look at the broader social, historical and political contexts in which such texts have been produced and read. The findings of interpretive and critical analyses of news accounts of medicine, health, disease and illness suggest that there is a wealth of meaning beneath the surface layer of texts. Common ways of portraying illness, or the threat of illness, in such texts often incorporate imagery drawn from an identifiable range of ideologies and discourses. These include the following: hygiene and cleanliness, war, invasion, fear, death, violence, heroicism, masculinity/femininity, elitism, contamination, vilification, blame, disaster/hope, uncontrolled spread/control, xenophobia, technology, activeness/passiveness, surveillance, and order/disorder (Karpf, 1988; Sontag, 1989; Haraway, 1989; Potter, Wetherell and Chitty, 1991; Martin, 1990, 1992; Hartouni, 1991; Noble and Bell, 1992).

It is no accident that such ideologies seem constantly to recur in news texts. Their presence suggests certain societal anxieties and concerns about gender relations and sexuality, about the domination of science and technology in western society, and ultimately, about the state's control and surveillance over the health and order of the body politic as well as that of the body corporeal. The textuality of AIDS as news lends itself to similar critical analysis. Far more than any other disease, illness or condition reported in the news media, discourses on AIDS have invoked stigmatization, discrimination, homophobia, racism, prurience, objectification, panic, a sense of emergency, moral meanings, and imagery associated with plague, sin, divine retribution, leprosy, and holocausts.

Dangerous desires

One of the strongest threads running through the subtextual layer of meaning in AIDS discourse in the news media has been the state's attempt to control sexual expression in any form not conforming to heterosexual monogamy. In Australia and other western societies, sexuality is a sensitive and highly repressed area of human behaviour. This attitude of repression is legitimized by the Judaeo–Christian tradition of regarding sex as sin. Despite the apparent liberation of sexuality as a topic of public discourse, it is still very much the case that such issues in western societies are fraught with mystique, shame, danger, embarrassment and taboo. Although in the late twentieth century masturbation, extra-marital and pre-marital sex and homosexuality have overtly been greeted more liberally, monogamous heterosexuality, ideally within marriage, remains the valued norm in popular culture, especially for women.

According to the socio-medical historians Brandt (1985, 1988b), Mort (1987) and Davenport-Hines (1990), sexually transmissible diseases have historically been subject to control based on moral grounds. Attacks on promiscuity based on medical justifications, then, can be viewed as stemming from the need to eliminate dangerous desires. Yet, because such attacks are couched in medico-scientific terminology, and often espoused by respected officials in the name of controlling fatal disease, the conservative moral values underlying such discourses are obscured. Such overblown threats, founded on the 'risk' of engaging in 'deviant' sexual activities, served in the late 1980s to create a needless and potentially damaging moral panic around all forms of sexuality (Bolton, 1992; Seidman, 1992; Singer, 1993). Foucault also singles out medicine as a major institution of the control of sexual bodies, whereby medical knowledge is inextricably linked to power relations. For Foucault (1978), the domain of sexuality is one of the most fundamental in the exercising of power over life in modern society, the subject of a web of disciplinary technologies and apparatuses of surveillance. Sex is where the disciplines of the body and the bio-politics of populations intersect. Sexuality involves both private actions and more public consequences, such as population growth, fertility control and marriage rates.

According to Foucault, matters of sex have not been repressed, but rather have been continually subjected to examination and discussion in a number of different and even contradictory discourses, which has elevated them to a level of extreme prominence by 'compelling sex to speak' (Foucault, 1978: 158). He suggests that rather than there being a uniform and constant silence on sex in the past three centuries, there has been a proliferation of public discourses which constantly refer to sexuality, privileging openness, liberation from repression, a return to the 'golden age' of sexual freedom, and which lament the silence on sexuality at the same time as they obsessively discuss and dissect sexual matters. Following Foucault, it may be argued that the very existence of regulatory discourses and practices around sexual expression serves to constitute dangerous desires as objects; indeed it brings them into being – by identifying them, labelling them, and constantly invoking them as needful of control. Just as the Victorians consistently acknowledged the power and presence of sexual desire (Seidman, 1991), contemporary discourses around sexuality seek to categorize, document and explain the varieties of sexual expression available to humanity.

In contemporary western societies, the popular media have had an integral role to play in the regulation of deviant sexualities, eclipsing that institution formerly devoted to safeguarding morals, the church. The proliferation and popularity of media products concerning sexual expression, of which 'confessional' talk shows such as *Donahue* and the *Oprah Winfrey Show,* and Madonna's *Sex* book are notable examples, support Foucault's observations that western societies are experiencing a proliferation of discourses around sexualities which seek to identify, categorize and examine sexual difference, and thus serve to constitute boundaries around a hegemonic sexuality which can be set apart from others as 'normal' and 'acceptable', determining the division between licit and illicit. The popular media act as influential agents in constructing and reproducing hegemonic visions of the body and its sexual activities. They face however a major contradiction in reporting sexual expression which differs from the norm, for difference is highly interest provoking, yet it violates the illusion that society is consensual. The trick is to titillate and then condemn, in order to satisfy the public's desire for 'utilizing groups as living Rorschach blots onto which collective fears and doubts are projected' (Young, 1981: 328). In this way, 'deviant' sexual acts are simultaneously publicized in order to satisfy the pleasure of prurient thrills and condemned to preserve the moral order.

Monogamous heterosexual pair-bonding has always been highly valued and greatly promoted by the popular media as the ideal state of existence especially and most overtly in advertising, teenage films and television situation comedies, where the importance of appearing attractive to the opposite sex and to attract a lifelong partner is

reiterated with monotonous regularity. The happy and attractive heterosexual couple is a dominant icon in consumer society; the homosexual couple, male or female, with the exception of specialized media
directed at the gay market, is virtually invisible. Even before the advent of AIDS it was rarely suggested in the media that homosexuality
was anything but dangerously perverse, 'sick' or alternatively, a source
of amusement although, according to Moritz (1989), lesbianism is
gradually becoming more visible and positively portrayed on American network television.

The news media constitute an important part of this categorizing
of 'normal' sexualities and desires. AIDS has provided the ideal opportunity to discuss sexual behaviours in explicit detail in public, in
the interests of safety and the provision of information. The urgent
nature of AIDS issues, due to the syndrome's high fatality and its
alleged potential to rapidly spread amongst an unwary population,
has forced western societies to confront certain truths about the
widespread existence of alternative sexualities, and to bring them into
open public discourse. The existence of homosexual and heterosexual
promiscuous behaviour as well as men's bisexual experiences has had
to be acknowledged, as has the existence of injecting drug users,
all stigmatized outgroups which in western societies are rarely discussed in the press in other than sensationalist and overtly moralistic
tones.

The arrival of AIDS, and the linking of male homosexual behaviour
to its aetiology, has demonstrated the thin layer of acceptance which
masks deeper anxiety and negative reactions to sexual difference. In
the early years of the epidemic, gay men became regarded as 'not
only deviant in their sexual habits, but a threat to whole humankind'
(Gronfors and Stalstrom, 1987: 55) because of fatal disease now associated with their sexual activities. The connection of gay men and
AIDS resulted in a slippage between the idea that gay men caused 'the
plague' to the idea that homosexuality itself was a plague (Weeks,
1986: 98). Watney (1989b: 75), for example, asserts that the response
to AIDS and people with AIDS or at risk of infection, is part of a
historical response to homosexuality in general, in which homosexuality
'is always available as a coercive and menacing category to entrench
the institutions of family life and to prop up the profoundly unstable
identities those institutions generate'. He sees AIDS discourses as
conforming to other western discourses intent upon maintaining social
control and regulating identity through such 'intimate mechanisms'
as 'sexual guilt, sibling rivalries, parental favouritism, embarrassment,
hysterical modesty, house-pride, "keeping-up-with-the-Joneses", hobbies,

diet, clothes, personal hygiene, and the general husbandry of the home' (Watney, 1989b: 82–3).

In the age of AIDS, the popular news media continue to represent homosexuality as undesirable√ In Australia (as in other nations), homophobia was most overt in the early period of AIDS reporting, when the 'Gay Plague' metaphor was at its peak. However the absence of gay men in AIDS reportage during the middle and later periods was demonstrative of a less obvious homophobia. Throughout those years Australian gay men were dying in their hundreds as a result of AIDS. Their plight was rarely given sympathetic press attention. The greater sympathy extended to people with medically acquired HIV or AIDS, and especially to children with AIDS, when compared to the representation of gay men with AIDS, was striking in press accounts. The overt homophobia of the early years of AIDS reporting had given way to an equally discriminatory silence about the mounting number of deaths of gay men, as simultaneously the deaths of a tiny minority of children with AIDS were publicly mourned.

Gronfors and Stalstrom (1987: 58) succinctly summed up public attitudes to gay men living with AIDS when they wrote; 'The history of AIDS has shown that there is a strong view that some people are worthier of being kept alive than others'. It has been observed by many commentators that western governments seemed very reluctant to fund research into AIDS when the disease was primarily limited to deviant out-groups, who were considered expendable by virtue of their social undesirability and the supposed threats they placed to social order. This sentiment has been echoed in public arenas: for example, the then Australian Commonwealth Shadow Minister for Health, Wilson Tuckey, at the Third Australian National Conference on AIDS, after quoting figures showing that 90 per cent of people who are HIV antibody positive are gay men, asserted that, 'AIDS is very much a disease that results from deliberate and possibly unnatural activity. You don't catch AIDS, you let someone give it to you' (Tuckey, 1988: 739). Likewise, an editorial published in the prestigious international science journal, *Nature*, spoke of the 'pathetic promiscuity of male homosexuals' as a risk factor for the spread of HIV (Anon., 1983: 749). Given the prestigious status of such forums of homophobic opinion, it is hardly surprising that news accounts of people living with AIDS have also adopted discriminatory tones, relying as they do on such authoritative sources to construct the news.

The 'AIDS is deviance' metaphor has proved powerful and long-lasting. The lexical formulae developed by AIDS reportage in the early years were still apparent in later press accounts of the disease, but had expanded and diverged into a greater number of contesting discourses. In Australia, even though the focus of news articles changed during the 'Grim Reaper' period of reporting to emphasize the threat posed by AIDS to the entire population through 'normal' heterosexual sexual activity, ideologies concerning sexuality and deviance continued to underpin press discourses. The dominant framework for AIDS reporting had been instituted: AIDS had been socially constructed as a disease of deviance. Even when children and adult recipients of infected blood products began to appear among the ranks of people living with AIDS, the cultural construction of AIDS as a disease of deviance had become so ingrained that these individuals were represented in the press in terms of how atypical they were of people living with AIDS, how they were 'innocent sufferers' in contrast to the guilt surrounding the original sinners. Binary oppositions of us/them, self/other, normality/deviance, and innocent/guilty were of critical significance in maintaining dominant definitions of 'people at risk from AIDS' and how they should be treated.

The 'Grim Reaper' campaign, like the British AIDS education campaign run a year earlier, attempted to manipulate feelings of guilt by making strong links between sex, disease, death and punishment. Although ostensibly appealing to the audience's rationality, the doomladen imagery of icebergs, tombstones and volcanoes images used in such advertizements served only to invoke and exploit irrational fears (Rhodes and Shaughnessy, 1990: 57). The icon of the horrifying figure of death chosen by NACAIDS to make its point was equally explicit in demonstrating the government attitudes towards sexual permissiveness. Watney (1987: 179) has commented that the official line of British advertizements warning against AIDS and HIV 'is clearly anti-sex, drawing on an assumed rhetoric concerning "promiscuity" as the supposed "cause" of AIDS, in order to terrorize people into monogamy'. So too, the hidden agenda of the Australian government's AIDS education media campaign was that of presenting any sort of sexual encounter that was not firmly within the realms of heterosexual monogamy as undesirable, and quite literally, life-threatening. The emergence of AIDS as a disease that could be spread through sexual encounters between men and women provided the opportunity for the government and the press to condemn the order-threatening behaviours of casual sex and marital infidelity.

The word promiscuity, used in medical discourse to describe multi-partnered sexual activity, became used in popular discourse to denote 'persons who wilfully violate the moral code, who lack self-control' (Oppenheimer, 1988: 277). With the advent of AIDS, visions of a 'new morality' gained currency in some quarters; as shown, the metaphors 'AIDS is a moral reformer' and 'sex is danger', suggesting an end to the easy and open sexuality supposedly engendered by the sexual revolution of the 1960s and 1970s, were dominant in press accounts during the 'Grim Reaper' period of reporting. At the time of launching the NACAIDS campaign, Ita Buttrose made assurances that 'chastity was now in and permissive sexual behaviour well on its way out' The press was eager to espouse such moralistic and puritan views; article after article, supported by headlines, editorials and letters from the public, decreed that AIDS was a sign that the sexual revolution must be over.

AIDS at the *fin de siècle*

Strong (1990) has written of the 'epidemic psychology' which can be manifested in the face of a major outbreak of disease. He remarks that like times of war or revolution, epidemics can potentially create an atmosphere of lack of control, catching societies up in an 'emotional maelstrom' which evokes strong feelings of fear, suspicion, moralization, irrationality, panic and the need to take strong actions. In this electronic age of rapid global communication, the mass media play an important role in transmitting such fear. The 'Grim Reaper' campaign and its press coverage was the response of a government and a society in the grip of a psycho-social epidemic such as Strong describes. Certainly, as demonstrated, press accounts of AIDS following this campaign were redolent with apocalyptic imagery associated with the end of the world, depicting society running out of control and the need for a new order and new code of morality to beat the scourge. Just as in times of war, individuals are asked to act for the good of the nation: so AIDS, depicted as an incipient enemy, had to be vanquished by means of extreme measures, both on the part of the government (by conducting a controversial and 'hard-hitting' AIDS education campaign) and on the part of individuals (by reverting to idealized behaviour associated with fabled pre-sexual revolution times).

Such a response is characteristic of a society faced by rapid social change: there is a yearning for a return to a supposed 'golden age' of order, decency, discipline and propriety (Weeks, 1986: 90). Showalter (1990) draws a comparison between *fin de siècle* discourse surrounding sexual crises and fears of the apocalypse which marked the late nineteenth century, and similar views expressed throughout the twentieth century. The late 1880s and 1890s were marked by sexual anarchy, in which the laws which governed sexual identity and behaviour seemed to be breaking down: femininity and masculinity were being called into question, the words 'feminism' and 'homosexuality' first came into use, decadence seemed rife and sexual scandals rocked Britain, one of the most notorious being the trial of Oscar Wilde in 1895.

> In periods of cultural insecurity, when there are fears of regression and degeneration, the longing for strict border controls around the definition of gender, as well as race, class, and nationality, becomes especially intense. If the different races can be kept in their places, if the various classes can be held in their proper districts of the city, and if men and women can be fixed in their separate spheres, many hope, apocalypse can be prevented and we can preserve a comforting sense of identity and permanence in the face of that relentless spectre of millennial change.
>
> Showalter (1990: 4)

In the late nineteenth century, it was syphilis that was viewed as constituting the divine retribution for sexual decadence, inciting moralistic discourses on the need for reform and a retreat from the liberalization of attitudes. It was averred then that 'one transgression, a single sexual contact, could lead to a lifetime of suffering' (Showalter, 1990: 189). The threat of syphilis was used to justify discrimination and prejudice based on gender, race and class difference. So, too, in the *fin de siècle* discourse of the late twentieth century, AIDS has come to symbolize punishment for sexual sins, to inspire rhetoric dwelling upon end-of-the-world scenarios and apocalyptic visions. The major difference is, as Showalter (1990: 191–3) points out, that AIDS is inextricably linked with male gay identity and homophobic discourses, while syphilis was more anonymous and pluralistic in its victims, although it was most often discursively located in the body of the prostitute.

While sex manuals in the late 1980s and early 1990s, including those for gay men, now privilege monogamous and long-lasting sexual relationships, framing casual sex as dangerous and even pathological (Seidman, 1991: 197; Bolton, 1992: 182), it is a moot point whether AIDS provided the catalyst for a 'backlash' to a 'sexual revolution'. Such a contention reduces the complexity and contradictions evident in public and private discourses on sexuality to a simplistic notion that one single phenomenon, such as AIDS, has the power to change deep-seated beliefs and understandings that are rooted in historical and cultural processes, and are themselves characterized by conflicting discourses. Whilst sex in the age of AIDS may well be considered more dangerous due to its immediate link with fatal disease, there are several historical parallels which demonstrate that the danger of sexual activity, whether linked to disease, pregnancy or marital breakdown, is not necessarily a deterrent (Mort, 1987; Davenport-Hines, 1990). Indeed, for many, danger is one of the major attractions of sex which does not fall into the ideal of the marital heterosexual partnership. Such sexual encounters which diverge from the ideal are more common in the 'general population' than is normally admitted in the media and other public forums, although few people are willing to label themselves as 'promiscuous', given the moral burden such a term carries (Bolton, 1992).

Feminist critics have long argued that the 'sexual revolution' of the postwar period did not release women from sexual subordination to men. Furthermore, a disenchantment with the ideology of sexual liberalism was evident in the late 1970s, well before the first report of AIDS, with critics from several different quarters counting the costs of hedonism, highlighting the emotional poverty of pleasure-centred desire removed from social obligations, and calling for a restored moral order (Seidman, 1992: 57 ff). Yet the discourse of sexual liberalism has remained dominant in public forums, as a perusal of mainstream magazines such as *Cosmopolitan* or popular music videos will attest. The public realm has become ever more sexualized, while the discourse linking sexual satisfaction with self identity and personal happiness continues to be expressed. There are thus competing discourses on sex in the age of AIDS which swing between advocating hedonism and sexual liberation in the interests of self fulfilment, and the condemning of any type of sexuality which takes place outside the bounds of heterosexual marital monogamy. The latter has taken precedence in the news media's reporting of AIDS, yet the former continues to be dominant in many products of the entertainment media.

Gendered AIDS

Commentators who have analysed media and medical depictions of women in relation to AIDS issues in countries other than Australia have noted the subtextual elements of misogyny, the pathologizing of women, the representation of women's bodies as sources of contamination and pollution, the portrayal of women as wicked seductresses and the dangerous harbourers of disease and death (Treichler, 1988; McGrath, 1990; King, 1990; Juhasz, 1990; Carovano, 1991). Women were largely invisible in the Australian press' representations of AIDS.

To some extent, this absence is due to the profile of people living with AIDS in Australia, for there are very few women with HIV infection or AIDS.[1] However, women are at risk of contracting HIV via injecting drug use and sexual intercourse with infected men. When women did receive the attention of the Australian press during the periods of reporting analysed, they were generally represented using several stereotypes: the domineering, matriarchal but chaste authority figure (Ita Buttrose); the passive, innocent victim of men's promiscuity (the women dying of AIDS whose stories were personalized); the partner in heterosexual activity who was responsible for enforcing condom use; and the grieving mother of children with HIV or AIDS. Lesbian women were rarely discussed in the context of AIDS, nor did prostitutes receive significant attention in the press; excluded, perhaps, because of their deviance and lack of adherence to the above archetypes.

However, while female prostitutes were largely absent from news media reporting of AIDS during the periods covered in this book, there was a case in 1989 when an Australian prostitute incited a moral panic concerning the rights of people with HIV infection. 'Charlene', as she identified herself, publicly announced in a television interview that she was HIV antibody positive but was continuing to work without telling her clients of her status and without enforcing condom use. A little-used section of the New South Wales Public Health Act of 1902 was invoked by government health authorities to incarcerate her for a time for 'the public good'. News coverage centred around her negligence in continuing to work, neglecting discussion of the role played by her male clients in ensuring their own safety. Such an emphasis on the prostitute's responsibility to prevent the spread of HIV rather than that of the client is typical of the western media's portrayal of female prostitutes in the context of AIDS; see King (1990) and Juhasz (1990). Because prostitutes are openly sexual and promiscuous they provide a convenient target for moralistic censure and victim-blaming in the context of sexually transmissible diseases such as AIDS. Conversely, as my own analysis has shown, 'good' women who are not paid for sex are viewed as the victims of promiscuous or bisexual men, and their youth and sexual inexperience is made much of in media accounts.

Contradictory representations therefore dominated press attention to AIDS and women. On the one hand, women were portrayed as vulnerable, unsuspecting, dependent, unlucky in love, falling prey to the devious sexuality of their male partners, denied agency. Those women with AIDS were described as losing their looks, wasting away, growing weak, but accepting of their fate. Suzi Lovegrove, the young and attractive wife and mother who was the subject of a documentary screened during the 'Grim Reaper' period of AIDS reporting, represented the archetype of the feminine, passive victim of casual sex. Conversely, the dominance of Buttrose as an authority figure in press coverage during the middle years of reporting, and the constant quoting of her exhortations that women should take responsibility for enforcing condom use, that casual sex was out, that celibacy is the best way to avoid HIV infection, ensured that women were also positioned as the moral guardians of heterosexual sexual expression, as saints rather than sinners, the vanguard of the new era of chastity and fidelity. 'Modern' women were portrayed as those who are able to take charge in relationships and demand condom use. In the later period of reporting, when the fear of heterosexual transmission of HIV had receded into the background, women were relegated to roles as concerned mothers of children with HIV or AIDS.

Representations of AIDS and women in Australian and other societies reflect dominant ideologies which problematize the sexuality of women in western society. Women struggle with competing pressures to perform sexually, to preserve chastity and their reputation, to please their partners, to maintain respectability, to avoid pregnancy and sexually transmitted disease, to bear children, and to juggle passivity and assertiveness. Discourses on AIDS highlight that the female body in western society is a fetishized commodity, constantly subject to the male gaze, and thereby amenable as an object of surveillance and control. The age of AIDS has ensured that an even tighter control can be exerted over the female body, with the twin ideologies of risk and patriarchy combining to foist the responsibility for instituting safer sex upon the female rather than the male partner in a heterosexual relationship. Discourses on AIDS maintain the female body as therefore paradoxically subordinated, disciplined, dangerous yet contained. These discourses are grimly ironic in a culture where women are not able to exert full control over their own sexuality, much less that of their partners (Patton, 1989a; Waldby, Kippax and Crawford, 1991; Holland, Ramazanoglu, Scott *et al.*, 1990, 1991).

It is also noteworthy that while heterosexual women during the 'Grim Reaper' period were highlighted as a new risk category, discussion of the specific risk posed by HIV to heterosexual men via sexual activities was largely absent. Heterosexual men achieved prominence in Australian newspaper coverage only by virtue of occupying powerful occupational roles in the public domain as government ministers, officials, doctors working with people living with AIDS, medical researchers and epidemiologists. These male news actors were active protagonists, seeking to fight against AIDS rather than passively accepting their fate like the women victims of AIDS. As shown in earlier chapters, male heterosexuals with AIDS who did receive news coverage were primarily men with haemophilia who had contracted HIV through infected blood products or, in the case of Geoffrey Pearce, a prison officer who had allegedly been infected after an assault by a prisoner with a hypodermic syringe filled with blood. Heterosexual men's sexuality as part of the private domain was rarely foregrounded, and certainly not to the same extent as was that of heterosexual women. The male partners of the new women 'victims' were mentioned as the route of their infection, but such men hovered in the background of personalized stories, shadowy figures of contamination, part of the victims' past lives and therefore no longer of interest. This neglect of representing heterosexual men as themselves susceptible to HIV infection through sexual activity, and the lack of reporting portraying male heterosexual behaviour specifically as problematic, reflects Australian government AIDS policy documents and programmes, which have routinely omitted mention of heterosexual men as a priority group for AIDS prevention, and have not attempted to persuade heterosexual men to reconsider their sexual behaviour (Waldby, Kippax and Crawford, 1991).

Body boundaries and fear of invasion

A curious result of the AIDS epidemic is the way in which the discussion of sexual acts and sexual secretions have had to be introduced into public discourse to an unprecedented extent, particularly in public health education campaigns. However, greater public acknowledgment of formerly unmentionable body products and processes has hardly relaxed society's opprobrium. In fact, because public health discourse has emphasized the 'unclean' and contaminating nature of sexual fluids and sexual acts, such matters have been regarded with as much, if not more, fear than ever before. The discourse of risk has served not only to warn, but to disgust. AIDS has thus become very much associated in people's minds with the control of bodily fluids; specifically the evil, disease-carrying, unmentionable sexual fluids of semen and vaginal secretions. These bodily products, already in modern society regarded with disgust, have taken on instrumental as well as expressive danger because of their undoubted biological ability to spread the new virus. Sex, now more than ever, is 'a risky business' (Clatts and Mutchler, 1989: 108).

At a deeper level of meaning, AIDS discourse has roused pollution, contagion and contamination anxieties to do with the maintenance of bodily and societal boundaries against invaders. Social mores which dictate the control of bodily orifices and their waste products are more to do with social organization than with the laws of nature (Douglas, 1979). The pollution ideas of cultures, the laws which govern the control of matter and determine what is 'clean' and what 'dirty', serve to reinforce social pressures: '. . . the laws of nature are dragged in to sanction the moral code' (Douglas, 1979: 3). Organic matter which is not intrinsically unhygienic but is culturally unacceptable is defined as 'dirt'. Hence the disgust levelled by western societies at sexual fluids, reflecting anxieties about sexual danger, about the assumed power of sexual urges (and in particular homosexual and promiscuous heterosexual urges) to break down the social structures which support existing social organization, such as monogamous pair-bonding, marriage, and the family.

Hence too, the anxiety around any overt social recognition and legitimation of anal sexual activity, which is symbolic of sex for recreation and not for procreation. Cultural notions to do with the uncleanliness and forbidden nature of the digestive tract dictate that sexual enjoyment should not be obtained from contact with the anus. As Poirier (1988: 466, emphasis in the original) has commented:

> The anus figures as the bodily equivalent of the dark centre of the earth, the place of insubordination and decreation ... Love may have pitched his mansion in the place of excrement in one of Yeats' poems, but Dante and the church fathers knew that the physical proximity of the seat of waste with the source of birth required that, *conceptually*, they be placed as far away as possible from one another.

Part of this response today is related to the means by which HIV is most easily transmitted sexually from person to person; penetrative peno-anal sexual activity. The anus has been labelled as the contaminated part of the body, and the emergence of the AIDS epidemic seems to bolster this notion, 'proving' as it does that anal sexual activity is unnatural and disgusting. When anal sex is male-to-male, the 'otherness' of the participants is further highlighted, arousing fears for heterosexual men of penetration by another, of being overpowered and 'taken', of losing control over the boundaries of one's own body (Redman, 1991: 25).

AIDS therefore invokes anxiety on two levels. First it violates pollution ideas, being inextricably interlinked with the containing of blood and sexual fluids in their rightful places. This fear can be regarded as arising from a rational basis, for such fluids are indeed physically threatening, carrying as they do HIV in concentrated quantities. Contagion and the threat of disease spreading uncontrollably are real and ancient fears for any society (Rosenberg, 1986). Less obviously, however, these pollution ideas are interbound with anxieties about difference, and above all, the need to control body boundaries. Hence the prominence of such metaphors as 'sex is danger,' and the binary oppositions routinely present in press accounts of AIDS referring to bad blood versus good blood, and to danger versus safety. In Australia and other western societies these fears have traditionally found their expression in religious laws, which dictate how sexuality should be expressed. Hence the quasi-religious tones of newspaper reports discussing the dangers posed by AIDS and the subsequent need to return to old values.

Several cultural theorists writing about AIDS (Treichler, 1989; Sontag, 1989; Patton, 1990) have noted the dominance of the discourse of invasion which has permeated both popular and medical texts referring to the disease. The discourse of invasion is most often framed in terms of the body's internal defences to pathogens. The cells of the immune system are frequently described, for example, as 'fighting' 'foreign' or 'alien' 'enemies' such as bacteria or viruses by 'mounting' a 'campaign' (Haraway, 1989; Martin, 1990, 1992). Bodies are visualized as being 'filled with tiny defending armies whose mission [i]s to return the "self" to the precarious balance of health' (Patton, 1990: 60). There is clearly a discursive link between the rhetoric of invasion and war which permeates news and scientific accounts of the effects of HIV at the cellular level, and the battle metaphors which position the 'ordinary heterosexual population' as fighting a war against the invasion of the deviant 'other'. Like HIV lurking silently within the nucleus of a cell, the 'other', the gay man, prostitute or injecting drug user, lurks within the body politic, breaking down boundaries by spreading disease into the heterosexual population using bisexual or promiscuous men as the 'carriers' of infection.

According to this discourse, the only defences are education, on the one hand, and medical science, on the other. Persuading mass behaviour change by means of media education campaigns seemed the logical strategy in late 1986 and 1987 when the 'general' population was thought to be at risk from AIDS. However, by 1990, once the threat to everyone seemed unlikely to eventuate, the promise of education as a weapon against AIDS began to lose its potency and the focus of reporting moved from attempts to change behaviour in a large group of people to the progress made by medical researchers in developing drugs to treat the much smaller group of individuals already infected, or developing a vaccine to administer to those considered to be 'at high risk'. Biomedical science was once again foregrounded as the major hope in fighting AIDS.

The rhetoric surrounding virology and immunology served to validate such a return to biomedicine as the best solution to prevent AIDS. The discourse of invasion by the foreign invader HIV and the threatened breakdown of the body's own defence system against such a wily aggressor conveniently constructed a horror story in which drugs and medical science could be positioned as saviours. Behavioural strategies were represented as 'simply stop-gap measures, only necessary until science "puts things right"' (Patton, 1990: 64). In Australian press coverage of AIDS, the metaphors 'Medicine as war against disease', 'AIDS is an enemy' and 'AIDS is a hidden danger' and the binary oppositions centring on deviance versus normality, functioned as persuasive rhetorical devices by which medical science was positioned as the best means of coming to the aid of the body when it had failed to protect itself.

There is a constant tension in such discourse between the responsibility of the individual to protect him or herself against disease (the 'education is the only solution to AIDS' notion) and the need of the institution of biomedicine continually to validate itself as deserving of continued support and funding. In press accounts of AIDS, this tension was often resolved by a discourse which conceptualized the body at different levels. The twin ideologies of medicine as saviour and individual responsibility for health could be successfully combined if medicine was represented as coming to the individual's aid when that person's 'army' of internal defences failed. Thus people whose immune systems were not functioning adequately because they were HIV antibody positive could be presented as failures on two counts: first, by allowing invasion of HIV in the first place (via the deviant routes of 'unnatural' sexual activity or injecting drug use), and second, by experiencing the failure of their immune system to respond to subsequent invasions of opportunistic infections, thus requiring further invasion by aggressive biomedical intervention.

The discourse of invasion has wider implications for the ways in which late capitalist societies view the body. It draws upon discourses which target the body as a site of toxicity, contamination and catastrophe, subject to and needful of a high degree of surveillance and control. According to this discourse, no longer is the body a temple to be worshipped as the house of God: instead it has become a commodified and regulated object which must be strictly monitored by its owner to prevent lapses into health-threatening behaviours.

Kroker and Kroker (1988: 10 ff) term the obsession with clean bodily fluids as 'Body McCarthyism', an hysterical new temperance movement which targets the body's secretions and which expresses anxiety over the invasion of the body by viral agents. The external boundaries of the body are closely guarded under Body McCarthyism, and the 'absolute purity of the body's circulatory exchanges [becomes] the new gold standard of an immunological politics' (Kroker and Kroker, 1988: 11). Discourses on AIDS during all three periods of reporting drew upon these anxieties, the need to define boundaries between 'self' and the 'other', to construct a *cordon sanitaire* between the contaminated and those at risk of contamination, to protect against invasion from without and within.

Moral threats and risk discourse

The linking of issues of morality, sexuality, deviance and control when explaining illness and disease is a cultural tendency which can be traced back before Christianity (Nelkin and Gilman, 1988). Watney (1989a: 67) has noted that the fact that AIDS is still regarded as a retributive condition 'speaks volumes about the extent to which pre-modern beliefs about disease causation can continue to co-exist with other more scientific understandings'. Poirier (1988: 467) has also commented that once a plague or a threat of plague gets linked to a sexual act of any sort, then the expectation of divine retribution follows. Even before the Christian era, plagues were almost always taken to be signs of the gods' displeasure for sins, often, as in the case of Oedipus, sins of a sexual kind. Turner (1984) argues that there is a close link between the sociology of religion and that of the body which has been little explored. He suggests that ideas concerning asceticism and the control of sexuality have moved from the spiritual to the secular realm, while retaining their focus upon morality and body control. According to Turner, the recent philosophy of placing the responsibility for health upon the individual, as advocated by health promotion practitioners schooled in the preventive health perspective, is yet another apparatus of social regulation and control, 'masked by the language of disease' (Turner, 1984: 214).

Modern theories of disease often contend that illness can be considered as originating from psychological weakness; a powerful means of placing the blame on the ill, or assigning the victims the responsibility for becoming ill and for getting well. There is a propensity in public risk discourse to function ideologically the same way; to blame the victim. Different types of illnesses attract different meanings. Sontag (1989) cites as an example the linking of some forms of cancer with a personality which represses emotion. In her work dealing specifically with the meanings of AIDS (1989: 112–3), she points out that diagnosis of AIDS or HIV infection essentially, in western societies, identifies the person living with AIDS as gay or an injecting drug user, who is bearing the punishment for living an unhealthy life. There is therefore a subtle difference between the blame apportioned to victims of other illnesses, and that apportioned to people living with AIDS. McCombie (1986) similarly has argued that the HIV antibody blood test is a powerful symbolic ritual, acting as an anxiety-reducing measure for those who are concerned that the virus is getting out of control, as well as implicitly acting as a tool for detecting sexual difference.

Illness may thus be designated as originating from either accidental or wilful 'deviance', the sick individual categorized as either 'innocent' or 'deserving' of his or her fate. As the preceding two parts of this book have shown, throughout the history of reporting of AIDS, Australian press accounts of people living with AIDS continued to draw such a distinction, particularly in their personalized accounts of people with medically acquired HIV compared with infected gay men. The metaphors used to make sense of AIDS in Australian press accounts seized upon these concepts of blame and guilt. 'AIDS as punishment' 'AIDS is a moral reformer' 'AIDS as crime' and 'Sex is danger' all stem from these ideologies, as do the binary oppositions punishment/ reward, guilt/innocence, deviance/normality, and crime/lawfulness.

The concept of risk is pivotal to discourses on dangerous desires. The word 'risk' as used in public health discourse has changed its meaning. No longer a neutral term, risk has come to mean danger; and 'high risk means a lot of danger' (Douglas, 1990: 3). Any risk is now negative; it is a contradiction in terms to speak of something as a 'good risk'. Douglas goes even further by asserting that risk, in modern society, has come to replace the old-fashioned (and in modern secular society, now largely discredited) notion of sin, as a term which 'runs across the gamut of social life to moralize and politicize dangers' (1990: 4). There is a moral distinction between the harm caused by natural causes and that caused by another or oneself. Risk is like sin, a 'predictive' concept, for it looks forward to dangers ahead, should one choose to indulge in participating in a risky activity. Unlike the old concept of sin, however, the modern concept of risk, like that of taboo, has a 'forensic' property, for it works backwards in explaining ill-fortune, as well as forwards in predicting future retribution (Douglas, 1990). The opportunity to blame others for their misfortune occasioned by risk discourse serves to ensure social conformity, acting as a technique of coercion and legitimating moral principles (Douglas, 1986: 56–60).

There are other ways in which public health discourses serve to victim-blame and impute moral meanings for risk-taking behaviour. These have been particularly prominent in media and medical discourses on AIDS. For example, the epidemiological tendency to categorize people into groups, to identify 'lifestyle' factors as causative agents for disease and illness, shaped the early cultural construction of AIDS and the defining of those 'at risk' (Oppenheimer, 1988). AIDS has been represented as both an individual risk, from which people must protect themselves by adopting safer sexual practices, and a societal risk, posed by those already infected to others. In the case of AIDS, sins and taboos are synonyms for risks: if an individual engages in sinful, tabooed (unsafe) behaviour, despite all warnings to the contrary, then he or she will be infected with HIV. Casual sexual activity, in this view, is morally reprehensible; deliberately bringing risk upon oneself for sexual pleasure which is not socially condoned. The rhetoric of risk in the public health arena has introduced this new moral meaning.

Sexual contact without a condom has become a new taboo in public health discourses on AIDS. However, despite the admonitions of safer sex education, the association of condoms with AIDS has resulted in contradictory discourses around these objects; see also, Gamson (1990) and Wilton and Aggleton (1991). Unlike AIDS, which has very few positive meanings and nearly all negative meanings, condoms in the age of AIDS have both positive and negative associations. The paradox that has strongly emerged in the print media's reporting of condoms is that on the one hand condoms signify reduction of sensuous pleasure, while for the moralists, they represent licentiousness. Although both are negative and detract from the safer sex message, the two meanings could not be more contradictory. Condoms in the age of AIDS have been inextricably interlinked with the need to contain sexual fluids in their rightful places. The meanings associated with condoms now more than ever reflect society's anxiety about 'matter out of place'. To say someone has AIDS is to imply that he or she is a certain type of person, socially and morally defined and labelled (Clatts and Mutchler, 1989). So too, by association, an individual who uses condoms or who wants to use condoms may be labelled and ascribed characteristics. The condom user could be considered sensible, modern and healthy, but also immoral, risible, and promiscuous.

The exhortations of public health officials and panic statements in the mass media of the dangers inherent in sexual activity in the age of AIDS do little to dispel sexual anxieties: they imply that bodies have become 'pleasure palaces first, and torture chambers later' (Kroker and Kroker, 1988: 14). AIDS discourse in the Australian press has drawn upon these prevailing notions of blame and sin, of risk as a moral concept, casting those who became infected homosexually, by promiscuous heterosexual activity or by injecting drugs as the villains who are worthy of little sympathy because of their irresponsibility. According to this discourse only those who acquired their disease medically or inadvertently deserve society's understanding, to the extent that they are awarded financial compensation because they had no part in 'allowing' themselves to become infected.

Risk discourse in the public health sphere serves the political function of allowing the state, as owner of knowledge, to exert power over the bodies of its citizens. In the case of AIDS, the state has taken on the role of ultimate producer of knowledge/science and health in its efforts to 'educate' the 'carnally ignorant' population (O'Neill, 1990: 335–337). The mainstream press in Australia has largely supported and legitimized these efforts of state surveillance over the private domain in the face of the growing 'AIDS crisis'. In Australia, the pedagogic rhetoric used by the government in its AIDS education campaigns, its self-imposed mandate to 'shock Australians out of their complacency' was little challenged by the press. As has been shown, the metaphors 'AIDS is heterosexual' 'AIDS is a monster' 'AIDS is an apocalyptic disaster' 'Sex is danger' and 'Health education as weapon' were used by both government officials and journalists to justify attempts to incite wide-spread panic, anxiety and fear among Australians and the adoption of a paternalistic disciplinarian role in order to enjoin 'correct' bodily deportment. These initiatives on the part of the state were legitimized by the pre-existing discourse of risk which dominates public health rhetoric, and which embraces the right of the state to intrude upon civil liberties to maintain standards of health (Sears, 1992; Singer, 1993). Risk discourse, therefore, served as an effective panoptic agent of surveillance and control difficult to challenge.

Summary

In this secular age, AIDS, as reported in the popular news media, is an allegory, a contemporary moral tale of punishment, sin and divine retribution. Above all, a continuing ideology of homophobia has permeated media accounts of AIDS, both in terms of overt discriminatory statements and in terms of the more subtle, but equally homophobic, marginalization of the plight of gay men with AIDS compared with other people living with AIDS. The analysis has shown that the Australian press is an inherently conservative institution, which has been generally willing to support state initiatives to engender a 'new morality' by stressing the dangers of both homosexual and 'promiscuous' heterosexual sexual acts. In the interests of preserving the health of the population, the news media have attempted to 'police desire' (Watney, 1987) just as vigorously as have state public health agencies.

Notes

1   By the end of March 1992, HIV antibody positive women comprised only 3.9 per cent of the total of people reported as HIV antibody positive in Australia, according to the bulletin of the National Centre in HIV Epidemiology and Clinical Research (Vol. 8, Supplement 2, 1992).

Chapter 7

Epilogue: AIDS as News in the Second Decade

In western countries, with a growing realization that HIV infection has seemingly been contained within small subgroups of the population, and certain geographical areas, such as the poor, working class districts of major cities like New York City and Washington DC, and cities with a high concentration of infected injecting drug users such as Edinburgh, the urgency surrounding the AIDS crisis has ebbed. In the early 1990s AIDS is becoming viewed as 'another intractable problem, like homelessness and drug abuse' (Kirp and Bayer, 1992: 381). It is now recognized that AIDS control should be part of a long-term policy rather than crisis management, and that the major issue for the state lies in providing adequate long-term health and hospice care for those people suffering from chronic illness associated with AIDS (Bayer and Kirp, 1992: 41–2; Street and Weale, 1992: 206). In Australia and elsewhere, concern has been expressed that public support for the provision of resources to AIDS services, prevention campaigns, treatment and research is flagging, and that as the second decade of AIDS unfolds, the state will withdraw much of its funding and its commitment to AIDS prevention and treatment programmes (Carr, 1992; Kirp and Bayer, 1992).

The observation that AIDS has become a stale subject matter for the news media has implications for the manner in which societal attitudes towards AIDS have changed over the decade since its first identification. It implies, for example, that AIDS is losing its 'shock-value', its social prominence as a major health issue, along with its newsworthiness and capacity to inspire metaphorical description. In some ways, the lack of metaphorical discourse about AIDS may appear to be a sign of increasing social acceptance of those at risk from infection. However, it may also signify decreasing interest in the issue, which in turn might lead to a decrease in society's willingness to commit resources for prevention activities, and to provide long-term support for those infected with HIV.

As AIDS enters its second decade, it is therefore likely that news coverage will continue to diminish in both intensity and quantity, unless a new controversy or dimension to the disease which is considered newsworthy emerges. As has been demonstrated by many analyses of AIDS as news, the choice of news actors or news sources has been an important factor in shaping the agenda for the public discussion of AIDS issues. These 'talking heads', or individuals sought by journalists as the subject of news or to provide opinions worthy of quotation, have persuasive power which is directly linked to their level of public standing or popularity. It is clear that medical expertise about AIDS, or personal experience with HIV infection is no guarantee of receiving a public voice in debates surrounding AIDS, especially if a person living with AIDS is a member of a stigmatized minority outgroup such as gay men or injecting drug users.

It is likely that the well-known will continue to attract a disproportionate level of media coverage of AIDS issues, especially if a famous person's HIV seropositivity is revealed. The death of British rock star Freddie Mercury in 1991 ended years of speculation about his HIV status and homosexuality. Australian Stuart Challender, conductor of the Sydney Symphony Orchestra, died in late 1991 after a public admission of his seropositivity and homosexuality forced by the Australian media's threats to expose him against his will. In April 1992, American tennis player Arthur Ashe called a media conference to publicly announce his seropositive status. Ashe had reportedly kept his antibody status secret for four years, but was forced into the public eye when the American tabloid newspaper *USA Today* threatened to publish a story about his illness. To avoid the stigma of imputed homosexuality, Ashe was careful to emphasize that he had acquired HIV through receiving infected blood products following heart surgery in 1983. He died of AIDS in February 1993. World-famous ballet dancer Rudolph Nureyev had died of the syndrome a month earlier after years of attempting to keep his seropositivity secret.

Although public exposure is traumatic for well-known figures living with AIDS, it has been suggested that the publicizing of their illness or death has had a positive effect in terms of 'humanizing' AIDS and people living with AIDS. For example, it has been asserted that Rock Hudson's death was a turning point in the American media's coverage of AIDS, for 'it gave the epidemic an emotional meaning that had not been conveyed by ... monthly statistics on the number of reported AIDS cases' (Rogers, Dearing and Chang, 1991: 14). However, the attempts made by many such figures to conceal their seropositivity or illnesses associated with AIDS, their reluctance to be publicly revealed as gay, or if they were not gay, their efforts to emphasize their heterosexuality, merely serve to reinforce the notion that homosexuality, and by association, HIV and AIDS, are guilty secrets. Few well-known people have wanted to face the intense media coverage and inevitable vilification associated with being HIV antibody positive. Furthermore, media coverage of AIDS which is based upon the pronouncements or lifestyles of public figures has, at times, drawn attention to discriminatory, distorted and homophobic views; for example, the statements made by the British peer Lord Kilbracken mentioned in Chapter One.

A more recent example of the importance of fame in renewing the news media's attention in AIDS is the intervention of the late Professor Fred Hollows in the AIDS debate in Australia in early 1992. Although he was medically qualified, Professor Hollows was neither an epidemiologist nor a specialist in HIV-related health issues. He was instead an ophthalmologist who has received acclaim for his voluntary work amongst Ethiopians and Aborigines with retinal disease. However, the respect accorded Hollows for his work (he was Australian of the Year in 1991) meant that despite his relative lack of expertise in AIDS, the opinions he expressed received widespread coverage in the Australian popular media. Hollows' entry into the AIDS arena provoked more interest in issues surrounding AIDS than any other incident that year, raising important questions concerning the 'ownership' of AIDS.

Controversy was initially generated in early March 1992 when statements made by Hollows first made headlines in the Australian press. Hollows had been invited to make the opening address at the First National Aboriginal HIV/AIDS Conference. He told the conference that Aboriginal communities would have to consider compulsory HIV antibody testing of all visitors and the quarantining of members of their communities affected by HIV to control the spread of the virus. Hollows also alleged that AIDS in Australia was mainly confined to gay men, and that heterosexuals had little to fear from HIV infection. These statements were considered newsworthy enough to be reported in the major metropolitan newspapers the following day, where he was criticized both by Aboriginal leaders who resented the suggestion that Aborigines were at high risk of contracting HIV, and by representatives of AIDS community organizations who questioned his suggestions that quarantine and compulsory testing be used to control the spread of HIV. Headlines such as the following appeared in response to Hollows' assertions at the conference:

PROF HOLLOWS WARNS OF PACK AIDS GENOCIDE

Courier-Mail, 3 March 1992

HOLLOWS SPEECH SPARKS WALKOUT

Sydney Morning Herald, 3 March 1992

AIDS EXPERTS ATTACK HOLLOWS

Daily Telegraph Mirror, 4 March 1992

HOLLOWS IN THE EYE OF A STORM

Daily Telegraph Mirror, 4 March 1992

HOLLOWS STANDS BY AIDS VIEWS

Courier-Mail, 4 March 1992

HOLLOWS TURNS UP HEAT ON 'REACTIONARY' GAY LOBBY

Sydney Morning Herald, 16 May 1992.

Current affairs television programmes that week featured Hollows debating the matter with representatives from community AIDS organizations. In these interviews and other public forums he accused the 'gay lobby' of 'hijacking the AIDS debate in Australia' and of 'cashing in on the AIDS industry' by 'fudging the numbers of AIDS cases' in Australia. Hollows captured the attention of the news media for several days. While the journalistic format of allowing both sides of the argument to be expressed by news sources was adhered to in the Hollows controversy, many reports framed Hollows more sympathetically than his detractors, by orienting the headline and lead paragraph to his statements, making him the active news actor to which others must react. The tabloid newspapers were particularly supportive of Hollows' comments, positioning him as a courageous iconoclast with the bravery to pronounce views with which many would agree, but have been reticent to express because of the fear of harassment from intolerant gay activist groups. For example, a commentary in the *Courier-Mail* (4 March 1992) began with the assertion that:

> Professor Fred Hollows is not the first doctor to claim that the homosexual lobby has hijacked the AIDS debate. He is, however, one of the few doctors to say so publicly. Others, including a former senior health administrator in Queensland, would say as much in private but resisted going so far in public. They feared, not unreasonably, the kind of response from the homosexual lobby that has already greeted Hollows ... delegates representing HIV-infected people walked out in protest: such is the commitment of some homosexuals to full and open debate on the subject. No doubt Hollows will be accused of homophobia: this is another common response by the homosexual lobby to people who try to raise these questions.

References to Hollows described him variously as 'the prominent ophthalmologist ... Former Australian of the Year ... the renowned eye specialist . . . the professor . . . the eye specialist . . . internationally known as an ophthalmologist . . . the prominent Australian doctor . . . a long-time campaigner on Aboriginal health issues . . . head of the ophthalmology department at the University of [New South Wales]', all attributions which attest to his medical/scientific standing in the community and his philanthropic achievements. By contrast, his detractors rarely received headline mention as active news makers, being referred to more anonymously as 'the gay lobby . . . gay community . . . gay activists and AIDS workers . . . white homosexual community' or 'AIDS researchers and community groups . . . government-funded AIDS bodies . . . AIDS council . . . other critics'.

Later that month Hollows re-ignited the controversy by making comments during a business luncheon in which he disparaged the National AIDS Strategy, alleging that education strategies were not working and that medical researchers and gay groups were profiting from receiving grants for AIDS research and education. Headlines again centred on the contentious nature of his claims:

HOLLOWS RENEWS ATTACK AGAINST AIDS STRATEGY
Sydney Morning Herald, 25 March 1992
HOLLOWS BLASTS 'BLOODY GAY LOBBY' OVER AIDS STRATEGY
Age, 25 March 1992
HOLLOWS ATTACKS AIDS TREATMENT 'RIP-OFFS'
Daily Telegraph Mirror, 25 March 1992
AIDS COUNCIL SAYS HOLLOWS IS MISGUIDED
Age, 26 March 1992.

Several articles quoted verbatim Hollows' comments that ' ". . . the things [gay men] do to each other are best kept to themselves and not spread around Australia because we are interested in controlling the disease and it's not being controlled"' (*Daily Telegraph Mirror*, 25 March 1992); ' "You know what they say about male homosexuals. They say it's the same as Down's syndrome – even the best of families have them"' (*Age*, 25 March 1992) and '[AIDS groups] were setting up "immuno-logical empires" and "making money from treating AIDS patients and setting up AIDS units"' (*Sydney Morning Herald*, 25 March 1992). Two days later, articles centred upon Hollows' decision to withdraw from further public discussion of AIDS issues, citing the harassment he had received from AIDS activists as the main reason, damaging his fund-raising activities to promote blindness prevention efforts in developing countries: '. . . "I don't want to be seen standing up in slanging matches with members of the gay lobby anymore," Professor Hollows said' (*Sydney Morning Herald*, 27 March 1992). Later he was to describe

gay activists as: 'a reactionary conservative group desperately protecting its own . . . its interests are sectarian . . . it will have to resort to
hooliganism and fascism and that sort of thuggery to achieve its aims,'
(*Sydney Morning Herald*, 16 May 1992).

Hollows' remarks were greeted with dismay by members of non-
governmental AIDS organizations, who condemned them as homophobic, ill-informed and irresponsible. However it was very difficult
for these groups to criticize him without appearing victimizing and
intolerant, both because Hollows was so renowned and esteemed
for his humanitarian efforts, and also because he himself at that time
was very ill with cancer (from which he died in February 1993). Over
the next two months, Hollows' intervention into the AIDS arena continued to resonate. Other prominent 'AIDS experts' entered the
debate, such as Dr Julian Gold, the director of Australia's largest AIDS
clinic, the Albion Street AIDS Clinic in Sydney, and a news source
who had often been used by the news media since the early years of
the epidemic. Gold made allegations asserting that Australia's national
strategy on AIDS prevention was not as successful as was claimed, and
that dissenters had not received due attention because of political
reasons (*Australian*, 11–12 April 1992). A series of feature articles in
the *Australian* drew Hollow's opinions into a wider debate about which
groups were at risk from HIV infection in Australia, with headlines
such as

AIDS: WHO REALLY IS AT RISK?

                                            7–8 March 1992

AIDS: HAVE WE GOT IT RIGHT?

                                            9–10 May 1992

REDEFINING THE AIDS RISK

                                            4–5 July 1992.

These lengthy feature articles, published by Australia's only mass-
circulation national newspaper and one of the more conservative
broadsheets in its weekend editions, raised doubts concerning the
virological tenets about the relationship between HIV and AIDS,
questioned whether AIDS is as great a problem as was previously feared,
and debated whether Hollows' comments about the 'gay lobby' were
accurate.

Compared with news actors like Hollows, people living with AIDS,
unless well-known for another aspect of their lives, rarely receive the
opportunity to speak about their experience of illness except in the
confessional mode. Paradoxically, science demands complex and intimate information from people living with AIDS about their sex lives,

but once this information has been obtained, the voices of people living with AIDS are no longer tolerated. While AIDS activists have sought to resist this oppression, arguing that 'silence = death' to demand public attention, '[t]heir words are only allowed as data, pathos, selfish complaints, politicizing demands for civil rights, and at the alleged expense of public safety' (Patton, 1990: 131). The Hollows case demonstrates that when such a well-known and respected figure dissents from current public health policy it is difficult for AIDS advocates to reset the agenda without attracting further damaging publicity. In this case, Hollows as the main news source was able to frame the debate, using such emotive words and phrases as 'gay lobby . . . a reactionary conservative group desperately protecting its own . . . setting up immunological empires . . . hijacking the AIDS debate . . . sectarian . . . hooliganism . . . fascism . . . thuggery' to imply a conspiracy on the part of a malicious, self-interested and intolerant group capable of resorting to violence to maintain its position. He was able effectively to define AIDS activist groups as exclusively comprised of gay men with shrill demands, to position such individuals both as victimizers (of himself) and victims (of their own selfish sexual desires as people living with AIDS). By virtue of Hollows' public standing, for the first time since the early years of Australian AIDS reporting, homophobic statements received prominence in the coverage of AIDS issues. Rather than targeting gay men for their 'dissolute' lifestyles alone, Hollows' remarks incited a public criticism of the attempts of gay men to act collectively to attract attention to their claims. News reports positioned Hollows as a lone crusader, fighting for a voice above the clamour of AIDS activist groups.

As this example demonstrates, a continuing difficulty for AIDS activists in the second decade of the disease is the need to insist that gay men are a high priority for AIDS resources coupled with the imperative to reduce stigmatization and discrimination. On the one hand, activists have sought to generalize AIDS risk by insisting that HIV infection and AIDS can affect anyone, regardless of sexual practice; on the other, they have been forced to emphasize that gay men are those primarily affected by the epidemic so as to ensure continued funding. Hollows called attention to this almost schizophrenic representation (and demonstrated his own confusion about the issue) by alleging that gay AIDS groups were dishonestly manipulating and exaggerating the numbers of gay men affected with HIV in order to attract funding. However, he also alleged that AIDS prevention activities were not effective, that as a result more and more gay men were becoming infected with HIV, and that gay men constituted the only group at real risk from HIV infection. On all fronts, then, Hollows was able to position negatively gay men and AIDS activists, drawing upon old and well-established homophobic discourses to describe gay men as profiting from AIDS while at the same time constituting the major victims of AIDS because of their profligate lifestyles.

The publicity surrounding the HIV seropositive status of basketball player Earvin 'Magic' Johnson, revealed at a press conference in November 1991, may have had the opposite effect by alerting Americans to the fact that heterosexuals *are* at risk from HIV infection. By the end of the day in which he made the announcement, the American National AIDS Hotline had received over ten times the usual number of AIDS-related inquiries (Brown and Basil, 1993: 1). The impact of Johnson's revelation attracted far more public attention than any mass-media health education campaign would have been able to achieve alone. Johnson maintained that he had not engaged in male-to-male sexual encounters, or injected drugs. He did acknowledge that by virtue of his status as one of the most popular American professional basketballers, he had sex with many women. Johnson attributed his seropositivity to one of these encounters. Because of his status as sporting hero in American culture, Johnson's plight received much publicity and media coverage in the USA (Maddox, 1991; Brown and Basil, 1993). Johnson is now in a position to act as a spokesman for people living with AIDS and a educator whose opinions on AIDS issues may be sought by the media and publicized across the USA. Johnson's role as a person infected with HIV through heterosexual contact may continue to have a significant impact on news media discourses on AIDS in the early 1990s. At the time of writing, other western countries, including Australia, had not produced an individual equivalently high in the public estimation who has revealed their seropositive status due to male/female sexual activity; it may be argued that the heterosexual AIDS issue will lie dormant in the news media in these countries until such an event occurs.

As AIDS enters the early 1990s, debates about the 'ownership' of AIDS seem likely to continue to attract media attention by virtue of their conflictual nature. If the trend towards the stabilizing of the epidemic in Australia and other western nations continues, human rights issues relating to people living with AIDS, their housing, medical treatment and care, will receive a low, but steady level of reporting in the western news media. The serious problem of AIDS in sub-Saharan Africa and South-East Asia will continue to be reported in western countries, but perceived lack of immediacy and personal relevance will probably serve to limit wider media coverage. Unless popular media coverage of AIDS issues is sensitive towards the situation of people living with AIDS, it is unlikely that social change in the private sphere will occur. If the news media do not see AIDS as an important and newsworthy issue then the interest and support of the general community may well flag. Apathy and complacency may dominate, and continuing efforts to maintain high levels of awareness may be thwarted. In the tradition of cultural activism, it is therefore important that AIDS interest groups and AIDS activists continue to be aware of the tenor of AIDS news coverage so as to be equipped to counter inaccurate and stigmatized representations of the disease, and to be ready to challenge the opinions of those who seek to take control of public debates on AIDS-related issues.

Appendices

Appendix 1   The press in Australia

Over the period in which the analysis of press accounts of AIDS was carried out, details of ownership and control of the Australian press were in a state of fluctuation. Between the early 1980s and 1990, for example, several of the newspapers referred to ceased publication or merged. Australian newspapers during the periods of AIDS reportage here discussed were largely controlled by two main companies, either through direct ownership or the possession of a large proportion of shares in the company: John Fairfax Holdings Ltd and the Rupert Murdoch-owned News Limited Corporation. At the time of writing (mid 1993), Murdoch's News Limited owns seven of the fourteen metropolitan or national daily newspapers published in Australia (the *Australian*, the *Daily Telegraph-Mirror*, the *Herald-Sun*, the *Courier-Mail*, the *Advertiser*, the *Hobart Mercury* and the *Northern Territory News*). The John Fairfax group owns three metropolitan 'quality' daily newspapers (the *Australian Financial Review*, the *Sydney Morning Herald* and the *Age*) (Australian Press Council, 1992).

During the 1980s, the national *Times on Sunday* and its predecessor, *The National Times* for a time appeared each Sunday, but the former ceased publication in 1988. By 1990, the *Australian* and the *Australian Financial Review* were the only daily national newspapers published, with the *Weekend Australian* appearing on Saturdays. Currently each major Australian city has at least one, and up to three, newspapers printed Monday to Saturday, with some newspapers publishing Sunday editions. In the periods of reporting examined, there were up to four major metropolitan newspapers published daily in Sydney; the *Sydney Morning Herald*, the *Sun* (now defunct), the *Daily Telegraph* and the *Daily Mirror* (the latter two of which merged in 1990 into a hybrid called the *Daily Telegraph Mirror*). In Melbourne, the *Age*, the *Herald* (now the *Herald-Sun*) and the *Sun News-Pictorial* were published daily, while Perth published the *West Australian* and the *Daily News* (now defunct). Adelaide published the *Advertiser* and the *News*, Brisbane, the *Courier-Mail* and the *Daily Sun* (now defunct), Canberra, the *Canberra Times*, Darwin, the *Northern Territory News*, Hobart, the *Mercury*, Wollongong, the *Illawarra Mercury*, Launceston, the *Launceston Examiner*, and Newcastle, the *Newcastle Herald*.

Owing partly to their concentration of ownership in a small number of large corporations and their reliance on advertizing for revenue, all of the above publications have a mainly conservative stance; the left press has not enjoyed widespread support in Australia, and most of its publications have been very short-lived (Bonney and Wilson, 1983). However, among the newspapers here examined, a distinction may be drawn between the 'quality' broadsheet press (including the *Sydney Morning Herald*, the *Age*, the *Australian Financial Review*, the *Canberra Times*, the *Australian* and the now defunct *National Times* and *Times on Sunday*), the first two of which are routinely rated amongst the top newspapers in the world; the tabloid press, which enjoys a far larger readership and circulation; and the provincial press, serving more regional interests in smaller metropolitan centres. The vast bulk of AIDS reporting has appeared in the first two categories serving the capital cities. Given their regionalized focus, the provincial press has rarely discussed AIDS issues and events, except where a local resident has been involved.

Appendix 2 Chronology of major AIDS topics and the number of AIDS-related items in the Australian press by month, July 1986 to June 1988

JULY 1986 (Items: 141)

- British pop star Boy George might have AIDS
- Australian AIDS doctor (Julian Gold) says cure for AIDS is at least a decade away
- American television actor Paul Keenan has AIDS
- Bedbugs may spread AIDS in Africa
- Australian prison officers prevent condom supply in jail

AUGUST 1986 (Items: 132)

- Biography of Rock Hudson released
- HIV type II discovered by French researcher
- Ryan White (14 year old American boy with HIV infection) goes back to school
- HIV found in African insects

SEPTEMBER 1986 (Items: 223)

- Australian television programme 'Hypothetical' screened, debating AIDS policy
- Increase in AIDS cases in Northern Territory
- British scientist says his experiments with monkeys could mean

a breakthrough for the development of an AIDS vaccine for humans
- Various other vaccines and drugs for AIDS and HIV infection heralded, including AZT
- Australian university study on gay men and AIDS begins
- Australian man is on trial for shooting and killing his wife because he thought she and her boyfriend had set him up with a woman to give him AIDS
- Member of the Festival of Light (religious) organization, says 'AIDS could be the best thing that has happened to the human race since the Black Death'

OCTOBER 1986 (Items: 262)

- Three leading international scientists claim that the AIDS virus was created by US scientists in the laboratory
- HIV is sweeping Africa
- Rock Hudson's lover has AIDS
- Sydney AIDS clinic starts clinical trials for drug (Isoprinosine) to treat AIDS
- Prince Charles' valet dies from AIDS
- Australian policewoman awarded compensation after a drug addict spat in her face and bit her
- Australian professor (David Penington) predicts that there will be 1000 cases of AIDS in Australia by 1988
- Freddie Mercury (lead singer of pop group Queen) has HIV antibody test but is seronegative
- AIDS is spreading among American children
- Aboriginal ritual customs (incision, circumcision) an AIDS risk
- Heterosexuals at risk in the USA and Britain
- Penington warns that injecting drug users will spread AIDS to the general population
- Advertizing firms briefed on government-sponsored AIDS education campaign to be aimed at heterosexuals

NOVEMBER 1986 (Items: 288)

- AIDS education campaign aimed at heterosexuals first officially announced by NACAIDS

- Penington resigns from NACAIDS
- In Britain a person who died from AIDS is sealed in a concrete tomb when buried
- NACAIDS calls for school education on AIDS
- Research suggests that cigarette smoking may induce AIDS in HIV antibody positive people
- Injecting drug users' risk for AIDS: a conduit for spreading HIV to heterosexuals in Pattern 1 countries
- Fear of AIDS curbs heterosexual Americans' desire for casual sex
- Visiting American AIDS expert (Michael Gottlieb) warns that 5000 Australians could have AIDS by 1990
- Australian man with AIDS rapes his 14 year-old daughter
- AIDS deaths in Africa could rise to one million
- AIDS is the plague of the 1980s
- Condoms as protection against AIDS

DECEMBER 1986 (Items: 295)

- Proposal for Australian identity card which shows HIV antibody status
- Heterosexual AIDS cases on the increase in developed countries
- Ita Buttrose (chair of NACAIDS) backs school AIDS education
- Hypodermic needles are made freely and cheaply available to drug users in New South Wales pharmacies
- Premier of Queensland, Joh Bjelke-Petersen, bans condom vending machines in that state
- WHO announces that vaccines against HIV are being tested in several laboratories around the world
- Queensland government launches radio advertizing campaign, advising young heterosexuals not to engage in casual sex
- A young Australian man who contracted AIDS from a blood transfusion is awarded $730 413 damages
- Heterosexuals in the USA are becoming afraid of casual sex because of threat of AIDS
- Shares in Australian Private Blood Bank (which stores blood of individuals for their own use) rise
- AIDS in Africa becoming a great problem

JANUARY 1987 (Items: 225)

- American Surgeon-General warns that 100 million people worldwide could die of AIDS by the end of the century
- Australian heterosexuals at risk from AIDS – AIDS no longer a gay plague
- Condoms advocated for heterosexuals and gay men to prevent against HIV infection
- American entertainer Liberace ill with AIDS
- NACAIDS campaign publicized
- British health education campaign launched
- Controversy over British Medical Association urging people who have had sex with more than one person in the last four years not to give blood
- Buttrose suggests that pregnant women in Australia may have to be monitored for HIV

FEBRUARY 1987 (Items: 372)

- AIDS a universal threat
- AIDS spreading fast
- Condoms and safer sex
- US priest hands out condoms at one of his services
- Need for AIDS education for everyone in Australia
- Death of Liberace
- Australian man with AIDS weds
- Private Blood Bank continues to prosper
- AIDS poses a threat to Australian heterosexuals

MARCH 1987 (Items: 740)

- NACAIDS' $3 million 'Grim Reaper' campaign to be released soon
- Buttrose announces that two million Australians are at high risk of contracting HIV, 88 per cent of whom are heterosexual
- AIDS deaths soaring worldwide
- Condoms and safer sex
- Education crucial in beating AIDS in Australia
- AZT
- Private Blood Bank

- Buttrose promotes celibacy as solution to AIDS – says the sexual revolution is over
- Companies are making money from vaccine and other AIDS medical research
- Aborigines at high risk of HIV infection
- HIV may lie dormant for 15 years
- Qantas airline stewards have HIV
- Dentists becoming aware of HIV risk
- Free needle plans for injecting drug users in Australia

APRIL 1987 (Items: 940)

- Grim Reaper campaign launched
- Everyone in Australia is at risk from AIDS, says Commonwealth Health Minister (Neal Blewett) and Buttrose
- Condoms and safer sex
- Need for AIDS education in Australia: represents the only way to prevent the spread of HIV
- Demand for AIDS tests on the part of Australian heterosexuals
- Buttrose says there must be a change in morality – chastity is now in
- Penington warns of AIDS affecting the brain
- Four Australian children infected with HIV after being sexually abused

MAY 1987 (Items: 629)

- Grim Reaper campaign
- End of the sexual revolution because of the threat posed by AIDS
- Condoms and safer sex
- Study shows that Australian teenagers ignorant about AIDS
- Old fashioned mores on the comeback because of the fear of AIDS
- Penington claims gay bias in NACAIDS
- Penington disputes contention that heterosexuals are equally at risk from AIDS as gay men
- Penington warns of risk to Aborigines of AIDS
- Blewett intervenes in conflict between NACAIDS and AIDS Task Force

JUNE 1987 (Items: 534)

- Threat to Australian heterosexuals of AIDS
- Grim Reaper campaign
- End of the sexual revolution
- Condoms and safer sex
- Twenty-year-old Australian policeman shoots himself for fear he has contracted AIDS after assisting someone with HIV at an accident scene
- Advertizing executive (Simon Reynolds) interviewed about his creation of the Grim Reaper campaign
- Third International Conference on AIDS held in Washington
- Publicity about 'Suzi's Story' – an Australian television documentary about a young woman who contracted HIV via heterosexual transmission and died from AIDS, leaving her husband and infected baby son
- American scientist (Zagury) trials new AIDS vaccine
- Head of WHO's AIDS section (Jonathan Mann) announces that as many as 1000 million people worldwide may be infected with HIV
- Tony Basten elected head of AIDS Taskforce, in place of Penington
- Proposal before NACAIDS to test job applicants for HIV antibodies
- President Reagan urges routine AIDS tests for immigrants, prisoners, couples planning marriage, drug users and people with STDs

JULY 1987 (Items: 539)

- Australian Governor-General (Sir Ninian Stephen) at WHO meeting predicts that AIDS will spread at a horrifying rate and affect Australian families
- Condom vending machine controversy in Queensland: Premier Bjelke-Petersen still opposed
- Australian professor (John Dwyer) says AIDS cure likely in 4 years
- Heterosexuals in Pattern 1 countries are changing their way of life and becoming less sexually permissive
- Documentary 'Suzi's Story' shown on television to enormous viewer reaction

- Jonathan Mann visits Australia for WHO meeting – predicts world could have 10 million seropositives by 1991
- Penington clashes with Buttrose about NACAIDS policy
- Australian teenagers at risk of infection, according to NACAIDS survey

AUGUST 1987 (Items: 514)

- Queensland universities condom vending machines controversy
- Australian Catholic nun says condoms may be needed to prevent the spread of HIV, and is condemned by the Catholic Church
- Queensland teachers not allowed to tell students about condoms when discussing AIDS – only doctors are allowed to mention condoms in the classroom
- British woman with AIDS from blood transfusion passes HIV to her three children vertically and her husband sexually
- American study shows that HIV is far less contagious than other sexually transmissible diseases
- Drop in incidence of sexually transmissible diseases in Australia is attributed to fear of AIDS

SEPTEMBER 1987 (Items: 369)

- NACAIDS launches youth working party and five AIDS information brochures
- Buttrose says Australian women must take the initiative in safer sex
- Condom vending machine controversy in Queensland
- Study shows many Australian bisexual men are married and placing their wives at risk from HIV infection
- Pope visits USA amid protest demonstrations from gays and people with AIDS
- Australian servicemen to have AIDS test under new defence force proposals
- Seventy-seven per cent increase in AIDS funding from the Commonwealth government

OCTOBER 1987 (Items: 248)

- Five prisoners die in a fire in Pentridge Jail as protest against moving of AIDS prisoners
- Story of Patient Zero – the airline steward who American author Randy Shilts alleges spread HIV to the American continent
- Condom vending machine controversy in Queensland
- Gay Australian servicemen found to be infected with HIV
- American study shows that heterosexuals are at a higher risk of contracting HIV than ever before

NOVEMBER 1987 (Items: 415)

- Grim Reaper campaign
- AIDS in Australian prisons
- Condom vending machine controversy in Queensland
- Patient Zero
- Australian bisexual men may infect wives
- People in the Australian armed services told to 'dob in gays'
- Australian police burn and bury car in which a dead man was found who had AIDS
- British singer David Bowie ordered by American court to submit to an HIV antibody test after an allegation of rape is brought against him
- Safer sex messages to be inserted in Australian pornographic videos

DECEMBER 1987 (Items: 135)

- American women fear casual sex because of AIDS
- Pornographic videos with safer sex message banned in Queensland
- New Australian health education campaign announced to be directed at young occasional injecting drug users (the 'Get Real' campaign)

JANUARY 1988 (Items: 289)

- Rapid increase in AIDS cases in Australia
- American study shows that frequency of sex for heterosexuals does not always determine risk

- AIDS crisis looms in Australian jails, warns Professor John Dwyer
- Australian Defence force recruits to be tested for AIDS
- Princess Anne makes discriminatory comment about people with AIDS at AIDS Conference in London
- Buttrose resigns as chair of NACAIDS
- HIV found to affect one in 61 babies in New York
- Bisexual married men are spreading HIV in Australia
- Australian insurance companies to request HIV antibody tests of their clients
- AIDS still a big problem in 1988
- Experts predict that AIDS will be the biggest killer of young men in the world by 1991
- Actress Elizabeth Taylor's daughter-in-law has AIDS

FEBRUARY 1988 (Items: 300)

- Increasing number of Australian injecting drug users infected – second epidemic/wave of infection predicted
- Medical research for treatment announced
- Tracing of people with HIV through blood transfusions proposed in Australia
- AIDS in Australian prisons a problem
- High rate of HIV in babies born in New York (one in 61 antibody positive)
- Ear-piercing discouraged in Australia because of fear of HIV
- Australian actress starring in British AIDS education commercial

MARCH 1988 (Items: 339)

- Seven children have died from AIDS in Australia
- Book by Masters, Johnson and Kolodny about heterosexuals and AIDS published
- New Australian advisory AIDS council formed from AIDS Taskforce, headed by Professor Peter Karmel
- Friend of Princess Margaret has AIDS
- Gay soccer referee with HIV is charged for bringing the game into disrepute by British Football Association

- Conspiracy uncovered to kidnap a Sydney businessman's 15-year-old son and inject him with HIV-infected blood
- Australian professor suggests that HIV-infected people should be paid to forgo sex to stop the spread of the virus
- Elderly Australian couple gets AIDS
- Famous American pornographic actor, John Holmes, dies of AIDS

APRIL 1988 (Items: 344)

- NACAIDS bus ads banned by state governments as 'indecent'
- Australian Medical Association calls for doctors to wear protective suits and for compulsory testing of all patients
- Australia's immigration policies do not allow people with AIDS into the country
- AZT trial in Australia
- Researchers find evidence that indicates teenagers are more resistant to the AIDS virus than other age groups

MAY 1988 (Items: 339)

- Ten-year-old boy is first Australian child to die of AIDS
- Australian Bureau of Statistics proposes to test participants in next national health survey for HIV
- Qantas allows cabin staff with HIV to continue working
- AIDS tests for immigrants to Australia proposed
- Media conference held by Australian AIDS doctors is told that an AIDS vaccine is five to ten years away
- Australian AIDS expert (David Cooper) reports the preliminary findings of a study which tests the combination of AZT and acyclovir for treating AIDS patients
- Furore over NACAIDS bus ads which show drawings of condoms
- President of the Australian Medical Association calls for all patients facing major surgery to be tested for HIV
- AIDS adviser to the Federal government (Tony Basten) announces a proposal for sentinel testing for HIV nationally (testing blood taken for other purposes)

JUNE 1988 (Items: 364)

- New AIDS strain spreading in Africa (HIV–2)
- Announcement of first overseas clinical trials on humans of a possible vaccine
- National Health and Medical Research Council suggests that heroin users should be given heroin to stop needle sharing
- Proposal announced to facilitate Australians' adoption of children orphaned by AIDS or infected by HIV
- Saliva test for HIV antibodies developed overseas
- Blewett announces that AIDS is the 'biggest problem since polio' at Australian Labor party conference

Appendix 3   Chronology of major AIDS topics and the number of AIDS-related items in the Australian press by month, March to September 1990

MARCH 1990 (Items: 244)

- Boycott of San Francisco conference proposed by several Australian and international organizations because of restrictions placed by the USA upon entry of HIV-infected individuals
- New York doctor gets out-of-court settlement after suing a hospital when she became infected with HIV after a needle-stick injury
- Australian Member of Parliament is bitten on wrist by an injecting drug user and fears HIV infection
- AIDS in Africa
- British scientist warns that swimmers could catch HIV from raw sewage pumped into the sea
- American study shows that sexually active college students routinely lie about their sexual history
- American actor Paul-Michael Glaser's wife and children are infected with HIV
- British mothers' eight children may be infected with HIV through injecting drug use
- American actor Anthony Perkins has AIDS
- Roman Catholic Archbishop of Los Angeles asks priests and nuns to volunteer to become inoculated with a vaccine against HIV
- Queensland Rugby League officials ban bleeding on the field to safeguard against spread of AIDS

- AIDS vaccine GP160 developed by an Austrian drug company is found to protect chimpanzees against HIV
- Life Insurance Federation of Australia says that rising claims by people with AIDS may force premiums up
- Australian government is criticized by non-government organizations for delays in making AZT available
- Studies show that fear of AIDS has led to a drop in the Australian incidence of sexually transmitted diseases such as gonorrhoea and syphilis
- Australian television programme '60 Minutes' broadcasts segment about bisexual men who are married and engage in risk activities for HIV

APRIL 1990 (Items: 323)

- Problem of AIDS in Africa
- US journalist Michael Fumento's book *The Myth of Heterosexual AIDS* publicized in Australia, provoking controversy about the risks posed by HIV to heterosexuals in Australia
- Ryan White (US boy who contracted HIV through infected blood products) dies in the USA aged 18 years
- Several AIDS organizations and individuals propose a boycott of the Sixth International AIDS Conference to be held in San Francisco because of USA laws restricting travel of people with AIDS
- WHO reports that the world has reported well over twice as many AIDS cases in the first quarter of 1990 as they did in the same period in 1989
- French researchers succeed in stopping HIV from reproducing in a human cell due to the discovery of an antibody against HIV
- Australian Teachers' Union calls for compulsory AIDS education in state schools
- Papua New Guinea will screen for HIV all expatriates contracted for work overseas
- Research shows most girls in an American college are not using condoms
- American fashion designer Halston dies of AIDS
- Two young Queensland boys with haemophilia are dying from AIDS
- American District Court judge suggests that all AIDS victims be exiled to Australia

- Actress Elizabeth Taylor's mystery illness rumoured to be AIDS
- Australian High Court judge Michael Kirby tells law conference that laws are needed to protect people at greatest risk from AIDS
- More than 100 Australian people living with AIDS who contracted HIV through infected blood products sue the Australian Red Cross Blood Bank and Commonwealth Serum Laboratories for negligence
- Seven-year-old Sydney girl, Holly Johnson, sues Red Cross and Western Sydney Area Health Service for damages after contracting HIV via her mother's milk (her mother was infected through a blood transfusion)
- Melbourne neurologist warns that the pin-prick test for nerve reactions could spread HIV

MAY 1990 (Items: 334)

- AIDS epidemic in Australia is waning, says Commonwealth chief medical adviser
- AIDS incidence is not rising in heterosexuals in Australia
- Study by Centre for Epidemiology and Population Health finds HIV-infection in the Australian population is lower than anticipated: between 12 500 and 17 000 are probably infected, and fewer people than previously expected will develop AIDS
- Australian Medical Association recommends immediate administration of AZT to health workers with needle-stick injuries
- HIV-infected prisoner is convicted in the USA of trying to murder a jail guard by biting him
- Australian Life Insurance Federation says that AIDS threatened the viability of superannuation funds
- New Zealand woman jailed for torturing a man she believed had transmitted HIV to her sexually
- Brisbane judge tells jurors in a murder trial to wear gloves if they wish to handle a knife allegedly used to stab a person with AIDS
- The problem of AIDS in Australian prisons
- New South Wales Minister for Corrective Services announces that prisoners in the state will be required to undergo testing but would not be issued with condoms
- AIDS activist groups criticize the Federal government over the composition of ANCA

- Report of American research study gives hope that the drug DDI is effective treatment for HIV infection
- Head of WHO announces that between five to ten million people are infected with HIV worldwide
- American heterosexuals join National Chastity Organization
- President of the Australian Medical Association calls for compulsory six month AIDS tests for all doctors and nurses working in risk areas, as well as for patients undergoing surgery
- Australian actor Jack Thompson appears on safer sex warning messages on X-rated videos
- Italian soccer player develops AIDS allegedly after colliding with an infected player during a match, causing general alarm about risks of playing soccer and other contact sports
- Australian research shows that one in ten injecting drug users is infected: researchers call for use of drug dealers in AIDS prevention programmes
- WHO announces that world AIDS cases top 250 000 in number

JUNE 1990 (Items: 471)

- Sixth International Conference on AIDS is held in San Francisco
- Australian epidemiologist reports at conference that epidemic in Australia seems to be confined to mainly gay men
- ACT UP members protest at San Francisco conference
- Conference is told that several Soviet mothers have been infected with HIV from their babies via breast feeding
- Australian researchers report at the conference about study showing that Queensland medical students are ignorant about some aspects of AIDS
- Conference is told that an American-developed vaccine which has been tested on mice should become widely available in two years
- Elizabeth Taylor addresses the conference
- Criticisms of Australian government's new education campaign (testimonials and 'vox pop' condom ads) by Australian Medical Association and Catholic church: suggestions that money would have been better spent in targeting gays
- WHO warns that rapid spread of HIV in developing countries means that it will be more widespread in the next century than previously thought: estimates that six to eight million people are infected worldwide

- Controversy over Western Australian police listing details of people deemed to be at high risk (injecting drug users and known gay men) on computer
- Australian Commonwealth Health Minister warns that there is still potential for a major sweep of the AIDS epidemic through the heterosexual community: says possibly between 15 000 and 20 000 people in Australia are infected with HIV and do not know it
- Hyperthermia (heat treatment) successfully used to rid people with AIDS' blood of HIV in the USA
- South Australian health worker becomes the first Australian to have contracted HIV at work by a needle-stick injury
- Five-year-old boy is awarded $37.47 million in the USA after contracting AIDS from a blood transfusion
- Mother from Queensland watches her two young sons with haemophilia die of AIDS
- Fred Nile calls a proposed Sydney nudist nightclub an AIDS exchange centre

JULY 1990 (Items: 461)

- Three robberies in Sydney feature use of syringes as weapons
- Controversy over Victorian AIDS Council advertisement for print media which shows two young men kissing
- American woman claims to have contracted AIDS from her dentist during a tooth extraction
- Egyptian mummies in the British Museum are to be tested for traces of HIV
- Australian government sets up special working party to look urgently at overcoming delays in the provision of new AIDS treatments
- Association of Catholic Parents makes submission to Queensland's Criminal Justice Commission that gays should be forced to wear identification tags in public or forced to have counselling, and that all gays infected with HIV should be isolated
- HIV is found in blood samples taken from a British seamen who died in 1959
- Eight Sydney doctors have contracted HIV from needle-stick injuries: Australian Medical Association calls for routine tests of patients before all surgery
- Mother in country town in Western Australia withdraws her

son from school after learning that a gay person with AIDS gave his class a talk on AIDS
- Homeless youth at risk from AIDS
- Melbourne store-owner is held up by thief with syringe
- Victoria reviews state murder laws to cover attacks with syringe containing HIV-infected blood
- WHO announces that at least three million women and children worldwide will die of AIDS this decade
- AIDS threat in Asia
- Australian study shows that Australian general practitioners know little about HIV or AIDS: many do not want to treat HIV-infected patients
- Issue of risk posed by AIDS to heterosexuals debated
- Sydney prison officer Geoffrey Pearce is stabbed with blood-filled needle by prisoner: waits for results of HIV antibody test
- Warders in New South Wales prisons strike and call for segregation of HIV-infected prisoners
- New British vaccine P24-VLP to be tested soon on humans
- Trial of Melbourne man for rape who refused to wear a condom when requested by his female partner
- Compound extracted from a Queensland marine sponge may provide cure for HIV infection

AUGUST 1990 (Items: 548)

- New public health education campaign launched directed at multipartnered heterosexuals
- National AIDS Conference and International AIDS in Asia and the Pacific Conference are held in Canberra
- AIDS in Asia and Pacific Conference is told that AIDS epidemic is sweeping Asia and spreading to the Pacific
- AIDS will orphan three million children by 1993
- Incidence of HIV infection among Thai prostitutes is high: Australian men should beware
- Cardinal Sin of the Philippines criticizes advocacy of condoms as preventives against AIDS
- Australian Governor-General publicly supports new education campaigns at conference
- National Press Club debate about risks posed by AIDS to heterosexuals

- West Australian Opposition complains about explicit photographs used in gay-oriented safer sex booklets distributed by the AIDS Council of that state
- Controversy over poster directed at gay men produced by the Victorian AIDS Council
- Holdups in Sydney by people using syringes: call for legal response to acknowledge HIV-infected syringes as a new weapon
- First British tests of vaccine in human subjects
- American researchers develop a synthetic molecule (CPF) that attaches to HIV and prevents it from spreading to other cells
- Seven-year-old Holly Johnson dying from AIDS: her father seeks publicity about her lost case for compensation
- Australian Medical Association calls for widespread community testing to determine the extent of HIV prevalence in Australia
- Australian person with haemophilia sues the Red Cross after he contracted HIV through infected blood products
- High prevalence of AIDS in Romanian children
- Two Sydney garbage collectors are jabbed by syringes when collecting garbage and are tested for HIV antibodies

SEPTEMBER 1990 (Items: 414)

- AIDS cases increase in Britain
- Incidence of AIDS in Australian women rising rapidly
- Australian study suggests that menopause might increase risk of contracting HIV
- Prison officer Geoffrey Pearce is found to be positive for HIV antibodies
- Debate over AIDS in jails, concerning control of prisoners infected and penalties for assault with infected blood
- More prison officers are tested for HIV antibodies after being subjected to attacks by prisoners with syringes
- Several prison officers in New South Wales resign because of fear of infection by prisoners
- Holly Johnson dies
- Premier of New South Wales pledges to tighten security in the state's jails to protect prison officers
- More holdups in Sydney using allegedly infected syringes as weapons
- Two more patients of the American dentist who allegedly transmitted HIV to a patient test positive for HIV antibodies

References

ABRAHAM, C., SHEERAN, P., ABRAMS, D. *et al.*, 1991, Young people learning about AIDS: a study of beliefs and information sources, *Health Education Research*, **6**, 1, 19–29.

ADAM, B.D., 1989, The state, public policy, and AIDS discourse, *Contemporary Crises*, **13**, 1–14.

ALBERT, E., 1986a, Illness and deviance: the response of the press to AIDS, in FELDMAN, D.A. and JOHNSON, T.M. (Eds) *The Social Dimensions of AIDS: Method and Theory*, pp. 163–77. NY: Praeger.

ALBERT, E., 1986b, Acquired immune deficiency syndrome: the victim and the press, *Studies in Communications,* **3**, 135–58.

ALTMAN, D., 1986, *AIDS and the New Puritanism*, London: Pluto Press.

ALTMAN, D., 1988, Legitimation through disaster: AIDS and the gay movement, in FEE, E. and FOX, D.M. (Eds) *AIDS: the Burden of History*, pp. 301–15, Berkeley: University of California Press.

ANDREN, G., ERICSSON, L.O., OHLSSON, R. *et al.*, 1978, *Rhetoric and Ideology in Advertising: A Content Analytical Study of American Advertising*, Stockholm: Liber Forlag.

ANON., 1983, No need for panic about AIDS, *Nature*, **302**, 749.

ASTROFF, R.J. and NYBERG, A.K., 1992, Discursive hierarchies and the construction of crisis in the news: a case study, *Discourse and Society*, **3**, 1, 5–23.

AUSTIN, S.B., 1990, AIDS and Africa, United States media and racist fantasy, *Cultural Critique*, **14**, 129–41.

AUSTRALIAN PRESS COUNCIL, 1992, *Annual Report*. Sydney, Australian Press Council.

BAKER, A.J., 1986, The portrayal of AIDS in the media: an analysis of articles in the *New York Times*, in FELDMAN, D.A. and JOHNSON, T.M. (Eds) *The Social Dimensions of AIDS: Method and Theory*, pp. 179–94, NY: Praeger.

BALLARD, J., 1989, The politics of AIDS, in GARDNER, H. (Ed.) *The Politics of Health: the Australian Experience*, pp. 349–75, Melbourne: Churchill Livingstone.

BALLARD, J., 1992, Australia, participation and innovation in a Federal system, in KIRP, D.L. and BAYER, R. (Eds) *AIDS in the Industrialized Countries: Passions, Politics and Policies*, pp. 134–67, New Brunswick: Rutgers University Press.

BAYER, R. and KIRP, D.L., 1992, The United States, at the centre of the storm, in KIRP, D.L. and BAYER, R. (Eds) *AIDS in the Industrialized Democracies: Passions, Politics, and Policies*, pp. 7–48, New Brunswick: Rutgers University Press.

BEHARRELL, P., 1991, Information or myth? AIDS and press reporting of heterosexual risk, unpublished paper presented to British Sociological Conference, Manchester, March 1991.

BEHARRELL, P., 1993, AIDS and the British press, in ELDRIDGE, J.E.T. (Ed.) *Getting the Message*, London: Routledge.

BELL, A., 1991, *The Language of News in the Media*, London: Basil Blackwell.

BENNETT, T. and WOOLLACOTT, J., 1988, *Bond and Beyond: the Popular Career of a Popular Hero*, London: Macmillan.

BERELSON, B., 1952, *Content Analysis in Communications Research*, NY: Hafner Press.

BERGER, P.L. and LUCKMANN, T., 1967, *The Social Construction of Reality*, London: Allen Lane.

BERRIDGE, V., 1991, AIDS, the media and health policy, *Health Education Journal*, **50**, 4, 179–85.

BERRIDGE, V. and STRONG, P., 1991, AIDS in the UK: contemporary history and the study of policy, *Twentieth Century British History*, **2**, 2, 150–74.

BIRD, S.E. and DARDENNE, R.W., 1988, Myth, chronicle, and story: exploring the narrative qualities of news, in CAREY, J.W. (Ed.) *Media, Myths and Narratives: Television and the Press*, pp. 67–86, Newbury Park: Sage.

BOFFIN, T. and GUPTA, S., (Eds), 1990, *Ecstatic Antibodies: Resisting the AIDS Mythology*, London: Rivers Oram Press.

BOLTON, R., 1992, AIDS and promiscuity: muddles in the models of HIV prevention, *Medical Anthropology*, **14**, 145–223.

BONNEY, B. and WILSON, H., 1983, *Australia's Commercial Media*, Melbourne: Macmillan.

BRANDT, A.M., 1985, *No Magic Bullet: A Social History of Venereal Disease in the United States since 1880*, NY: OUP.

BRANDT, A.M., 1988a, AIDS and metaphor: toward the social meaning of epidemic disease, *Social Research*, **55**, 3, 413–32.

BRANDT, A.M., 1988b, AIDS, from social history to social policy, in FEE, E. and FOX, D.M. (Eds) *AIDS: the Burdens of History*, pp. 147–71, Berkeley: University of California Press.

BRANDT, A.M., 1991, Emerging themes in the history of medicine, *Milbank Memorial Quarterly*, **69**, 2, 199–214.

BRAY, F. and CHAPMAN, S., 1991, Community knowledge, attitudes and media recall about AIDS, Sydney 1988 and 1989, *Australian Journal of Public Health*, **15**, 2, 107–13.

BROWN, W.J. and BASIL, M.D., 1993, Impact of the 'Magic Johnson' news story on AIDS prevention, unpublished paper presented at the 43rd International Communication Association Conference, May 1993, Washington DC.

CARDUCCI, A., FRASCA, M., MATTEELLI, M. *et al.*, 1990, AIDS information and Italian youth: a survey on military recruits, *AIDS Education and Prevention*, **2**, 3, 181–90.

CAROVANO, K., 1991, More than mothers and whores: redefining the AIDS prevention needs of women, *International Journal of Health Services*, **21**, 1, 131–42.

CARR, A., 1992, More bang for the buck: dollars and sense in HIV/AIDS prevention, *National AIDS Bulletin*, **6**, 2, 8–10.

CARTER, E., 1989, AIDS and critical practice: reflections from the ICA Conference, in CARTER, E. and WATNEY, S. (Eds) *Taking Liberties*, pp. 59–68, London: Serpent's Tail.

C.D.C. TASKFORCE, 1982, Epidemiologic aspects of the current outbreak of Kaposi's sarcoma and opportunistic infections, *New England Journal of Medicine*, **306**, 248–52.

CHIN, J., 1990, Global estimates of AIDS cases and HIV infections, 1990, *AIDS*, **4**, supp. 1, S277–83.

CLARKE, J.N., 1991, Media portrayal of disease from the medical, political economy, and life-style perspectives, *Qualitative Health Research*, **1**, 3, 287–308.

CLARKE, J.N., 1992, Cancer, heart disease, and AIDS: what do the media tell us about these diseases?, *Health Communication*, **4**, 2, 105–20.

CLATTS, M.C. and MUTCHLER, K.M., 1989, AIDS and the dangerous other: metaphors of sex and deviance in the representation of disease, *Medical Anthropology*, **10**, 105–14.

COLBY, D.C. and COOK, T.E., 1991, Epidemics and agendas: the politics of nightly news coverage of AIDS, *Journal of Health Politics, Policy and Law*, **16**, 2, 215–49.

COMMONWEALTH DEPARTMENT of COMMUNITY SERVICES and HEALTH, 1988, *AIDS, A Time to Care, A Time to Act: Towards a Strategy for Australians*, Canberra, Australian Government Publishing Service.

CONNELL, I. and MILLS, A., 1985, Text, discourse and mass communication, in VAN DIJK, T.A. (Ed.) *Discourse and Communication*, pp. 26–43, Berlin: Walter de Gruyter.

COOK, T.E. and COLBY, D.C., 1992, The mass-mediated epidemic: the politics of AIDS on the nightly network news, in FEE, E. and FOX, D.M. (Eds) *AIDS: the Making of a Chronic Disease*, pp. 84–122, Berkeley: University of California Press.

CRAWFORD, J., KIPPAX, S., and TULLOCH, J., 1992, *Appraisal of the National AIDS Education Campaign*, Canberra, Commonwealth Department of Health, Housing and Community Services.

CRIMP, D., 1989a, How to have promiscuity in an epidemic, in CRIMP, D. (Ed.) *AIDS: Cultural Analysis, Cultural Activism*, pp. 237–71, Cambridge, Massachusetts: MIT Press.

CRIMP, D. (Ed.), 1989b, *AIDS: Cultural Analysis, Cultural Activism*, Cambridge, Massachussetts: MIT Press.

CRIMP, D., 1992, Portraits of people with AIDS, in GROSSBERG, L., NELSON, C. and TREICHLER, P.A. (Eds) *Cultural Studies*, pp. 117–30, NY: Routledge.

CUNNINGHAM, I., 1989, The public controversies of AIDS in Puerto Rico, *Social Science and Medicine*, **29**, 4, 545–53.

CURRAN, J., 1990, The new revisionism in mass communication research: a reappraisal, *European Journal of Communication*, **5**, 135–64.

DADA, M., 1990, Race and the AIDS agenda, in BOFFIN, T. and GUPTA, S. (Eds) *Ecstatic Antibodies: Resisting the AIDS Mythology*, pp. 85–95, London: Rivers Oram Press.

DAVENPORT-HINES, R., 1990, *Sex, Death and Punishment: Attitudes to Sex and Sexuality in Britain since the Renaissance*, London: Collins.

DEARING, J.W., 1992, Foreign blood and domestic policies: the issue of AIDS in Japan, in FEE, E. and FOX, D.M. (Eds) *AIDS: the Making of a Chronic Disease*, pp. 326–46, Berkeley: University of California Press.

DOLAN, R., CORBER, S. and ZACOUR, R., 1990, A survey of knowledge and attitudes with regard to AIDS among grade 7 and 8 students in Ottawa-Carleton, *Canadian Journal of Public Health*, **81**, 135–8.

DOUGLAS, M., 1979, *Purity and Danger: An Analysis of the Concepts of Pollution and Taboo*, London, Routledge and Kegan Paul.

DOUGLAS, M., 1986, *Risk Acceptability According to the Social Sciences*, London, Routledge and Kegan Paul.

DOUGLAS, M., 1990, Risk as a forensic resource, *Daedalus*, Fall, 1–16.

FAIRCLOUGH, N., 1992, Discourse and text: linguistic and intertextual analysis within discourse analysis, *Discourse and Society*, **3**, 2, 193–217.

FISHMAN, M., 1980, *Manufacturing the News*, Austin: University of Texas Press.

FOUCAULT, M., 1978, *The History of Sexuality: Volume 1*, London: Penguin.

FOWLER, R., 1991, *Language in the News*, London: Routledge.

FRENCH, R., 1986, *Mossies Could Spread AIDS: Australian Media References on AIDS, 1981–1985*, Sydney: Gay Media Group.

GALBRAITH, L., 1992, AIDS: how the gay press told the story, *National AIDS Bulletin*, **6**, 6, 18–21.

GALTUNG, J. and RUGE, M., 1981, Structuring and selecting news, in COHEN, S. and YOUNG, J. (Eds) *The Manufacture of News: Social Problems, Deviance and Mass Media* (revised), pp. 52–63, London: Constable.

GAMSON, J., 1990, Rubber wars: struggles over the condom in the United States, *Journal of the History of Sexuality*, **1**, 2, 262–82.

GILMAN, S.L., 1989, AIDS and syphilis: the iconography of disease, in CRIMP, D. (Ed.) *AIDS: Cultural Analysis, Cultural Activism*, pp. 87–108, Massachusetts: MIT Press.

GREENBERG, M. and WARTENBERG, D., 1991, Newspaper coverage of cancer clusters, *Health Education Quarterly*, **18**, 3, 363–74.

GRIMSHAW, J., 1987, Being HIV antibody positive, *British Medical Journal*, **295**, 256–7.

GRONFORS, M. and STALSTROM, O., 1987, Power, prestige, profit: AIDS and the oppression of homosexual people, *Acta Sociologica*, **30**, 1, 53–66.

GROVER, J.Z., 1989, AIDS: keywords, in CRIMP, D. (Ed.) *AIDS: Cultural Analysis, Cultural Activism*, pp. 17–30, Cambridge, Massachusetts: MIT Press.

GROVER, J.Z., 1992a, AIDS, keywords, and cultural work, in GROSSBERG, L., NELSON, C. and TREICHLER, P.A. (Eds) *Cultural Studies*, pp. 227–33, NY: Routledge.

GROVER, J.Z., 1992b, Visible lesions: images of the PWA in America, in Miller, J. (Ed.) *Fluid Exchanges: Artists and Critics in the AIDS Crisis*, pp. 23–51, Toronto: University of Toronto Press.

GRUBE, A. and BOEHME-DUERR, K., 1988, AIDS in international news magazines, *Journalism Quarterly*, **65**, 3, 686–9.

HALL, S., 1980, Encoding/decoding, in HALL, S., HOBSON, D., LOWE, A. *et al.* (Eds) *Culture, Media, Language*, pp. 128–38, London: Hutchinson.

HALL, S., 1992, Cultural studies and its theoretical legacies, in GROSSBERG,

L., NELSON, C. and TREICHLER, P.A. (Eds) *Cultural Studies*, pp. 277–85, NY: Routledge.

HALL, S., CRITCHER, C., JEFFERSON, J. *et al.*, 1982, *Policing the Crisis: Mugging, the State, and Law and Order*, 5th Edn, London: McMillan.

HAMMONDS, E., 1986, Race, sex, AIDS: the construction of 'Other', *Radical America*, **20**, 6, 28–36.

HARAWAY, D., 1989, The biopolitics of postmodern bodies: determinations of self in immune system discourse, *Differences*, **1**, 1, 3–44.

Hartouni, V., 1991, Containing women: reproductive discourse in the 1980s, in PENLEY, C. and ROSS, A. (Eds) *Technoculture*, pp. 27–56, Minneapolis: University of Minnesota Press.

HERLITZ, C. and BRORSSON, B., 1990, AIDS in the minds of Swedish people, 1986–1989, *AIDS*, **4**, 1011–18.

HERZLICH, C. and PIERRET, J., 1989, The construction of a social phenomenon: AIDS in the French press, *Social Science and Medicine*, **29**, 2, 1235–42.

HOLLAND, J., RAMAZANOGLU, C., SCOTT, S., *et al.*, 1990, Sex, gender and power: young women's sexuality in the shadow of AIDS, *Sociology of Health and Illness*, **12**, 3, 336–50.

HOLLAND, J., RAMAZANOGLU, C., SCOTT, S., *et al.*, 1991, Between embarrassment and trust: young women and the diversity of condom use, in AGGLETON, P., HART, G. and DAVIES, P. (Eds) *AIDS: Responses, Interventions and Care*, pp. 127–48, London: Falmer.

HUGHEY, J.D., NORTON, R.W. and SULLIVAN-NORTON, C., 1989, Insidious metaphors and the changing meaning of AIDS, *AIDS and Public Policy Journal*, **4**, 1, 56–67.

JENSEN, K.B., 1991, Introduction: the qualitative turn, in JENSEN, K.B. and JANKOWSKI, N.W. (Eds) *A Handbook of Qualitative Methodologies for Mass Communication Research*, pp. 1–11, London: Routledge.

JONES, J.W., 1992, Discourses on and of AIDS in West Germany, 1986–90, *Journal of the History of Sexuality*, **2**, 3, 439–68.

JUHASZ, A., 1990, The contained threat: women in mainstream AIDS documentary, *Journal of Sex Research*, **27**, 1, 25–46.

KALDOR, J., McDONALD, A.M., BLUMER, C.E. *et al.*, 1993, The acquired immunodeficiency syndrome in Australia: incidence 1982–1991, *Medical Journal of Australia*, **158**, 10–20.

KARPF, A., 1988, *Doctoring the Media: the Reporting of Health and Medicine*, London: Routledge.

KING, D., 1990, 'Prostitutes as pariah in the age of AIDS': a content analysis of coverage of women prostitutes in the *New York Times* and the *Washington Post* September 1985–April 1988, *Women and Health*, **16**, 3/4, 155–76.

KIPPAX, S., CRAWFORD, J., WALDBY, C., *et al.*, 1990, Women negotiating heterosex: a study using memory-work, *Women's Studies International Forum*, **13**, 6, 533–42.

KIRP, D.L. and BAYER, R., 1992, The second decade of AIDS: the end of exceptionalism?, in KIRP, D.L. and BAYER, R. (Eds) *AIDS in the Industrialized Democracies: Passions, Politics, and Policies*, pp. 361–84, New Brunswick: Rutgers University Press.

KITZINGER, J., 1990, Audience understandings of AIDS media messages: a discussion of methods, *Sociology of Health and Illness*, **12**, 3, 320–35.

KITZINGER, J. and MILLER, D., 1991, *In Black and White: a Preliminary Report on the Role of the Media in Audience Understandings of 'African AIDS'*. Glasgow: AIDS Media Research Project.

KLAIDMAN, S., 1990, How well the media report health risk, *Daedalus*, Fall, 119–32.

KLAIDMAN, S., 1991, *Health in the Headlines: the Stories Behind the Stories*, NY: OUP.

KRESS, G., 1985, *Linguistic Processes in Socio-Cultural Practice*, Victoria: Deakin University Press.

KROKER, A. and KROKER, M., 1988, Panic sex in America, in KROKER, A. and KROKER, M. (Eds) *Body Invaders: Sexuality and the Postmodern Condition*, pp. 1–18, London: Macmillan Education.

LAKOFF, G. and JOHNSON, M., 1981, Conceptual metaphor in everyday language, in JOHNSON, M. (Ed.) *Philosophical Perspectives on Metaphor*, pp. 286–328, Minneapolis: University of Minnesota Press.

MADDOX, J., 1991, Basketball, AIDS and education, *Nature*, **354**, 103.

MARSHALL, S., 1990, Picturing deviancy, in BOFFIN, T. and GUPTA, S. (Eds) *Ecstatic Antibodies: Resisting the AIDS Mythology*, pp. 19–36, London: Rivers Oram Press.

MARTIN, E., 1990, Toward an anthropology of immunology: the body as nation state, *Medical Anthropology Quarterly*, **4**, 4, 410–26.

MARTIN, E., 1992, Body narratives, body boundaries, in GROSSBERG, L., NELSON, C. and TREICHLER, P.A. (Eds) *Cultural Studies*, pp. 409–23, NY: Routledge.

MASTERS, W.H., JOHNSON, V.E. and KOLODNY, R.C., 1988, *Crisis: Heterosexual Behaviour in the Age of AIDS*, London: Grafton.

MATICKA-TYNDALE, E., 1992, Social construction of HIV transmission and prevention among heterosexual young adults, *Social Problems*, **39**, 3, 238–52.

McCOMBIE, S., 1986, The cultural impact of the 'AIDS' test: the American experience, *Social Science and Medicine*, **23**, 5, 455–9.

McGRATH, R., 1990, Dangerous liaisons: health, disease and representation, in BOFFIN, T. and GUPTA, S. (Eds) *Ecstatic Antibodies:*

Resisting the AIDS Mythology, pp. 142–55, London: Rivers Oram Press.

MEYER, P., 1990, News media responsiveness to public health, in ATKIN, C. and WALLACK, L. (Eds) *Mass Communication and Public Health: Complexities and Conflicts*, pp. 53–9, Newbury Park: Sage.

MORITZ, M.J., 1989, American television discovers gay women: the changing context of programming decisions at the networks, *Journal of Communication Inquiry*, **13**, 2, 62–74.

MORLEY, D., 1992, *Television, Audiences and Cultural Studies*, London: Routledge.

MORT, F., 1987, *Dangerous Sexualities: Medico-Moral Politics in England Since 1830*, London: Routledge and Kegan Paul.

MORTLET, A., GUINAN, J.J., DIEFENTHALER, I., *et al.*, 1988, The impact of the 'Grim Reaper' national AIDS educational campaign on the Albion Street (AIDS) Centre and the AIDS hotline, *Medical Journal of Australia*, **148**, 282–6.

MURRAY, J., 1991, Bad press: representations of AIDS in the media *Cultural Studies from Birmingham*, **1**, 29–51.

NATIONAL CENTRE IN HIV EPIDEMIOLOGY AND CLINICAL RESEARCH, 1993, *Australian HIV Surveillance Report*, **9**, 2, Sydney.

NELKIN, D., 1987, *Selling Science: How the Press Covers Science and Technology*, NY: WH Freeman.

NELKIN, D., 1991, AIDS and the news media, *Milbank Quarterly*, **69**, 2, 293–307.

NELKIN, D. and GILMAN, S.L., 1988, Placing blame for devastating disease, *Social Research*, **55**, 3, 361–78.

NELSON, C., TREICHLER, P.A. and GROSSBERG, L., 1992, Cultural studies: an introduction, in GROSSBERG, L., NELSON, C. and TREICHLER, P.A. (Eds) *Cultural Studies*, pp. 1–16, NY: Routledge.

NICOLSON, M. and McLAUGHLIN, C., 1987, Social constructionism and medical sociology: a reply to M.R. BURY, *Sociology of Health and Illness*, **9**, 2, 107–27.

NOBLE, C. and BELL, P., 1992, Reproducing women's nature, media constructions of IVF and related issues, *Australian Journal of Social Issues*, **27**, 1, 17–30.

O'NEILL, J., 1990, AIDS as a globilizing panic, *Theory, Culture and Society*, **7**, 329–42.

OPPENHEIMER, G.M., 1988, In the eye of the storm: the epidemiological construction of AIDS, in FEE, E. and FOX, D.M. (Eds) *AIDS: the Burdens of History*, pp. 267–300, Berkeley: University of California Press.

PARKER, I., 1992, *Discourse Dynamics: Critical Analysis for Social and Individual Psychology*, London: Routledge.

PATTON, C., 1989a, Resistance and the erotic, in AGGLETON, P., HART, G. and DAVIES, P. (Eds) *AIDS: Social Representations, Social Practices*, Basingstoke: Falmer.

PATTON, C., 1989b, The AIDS industry: construction of 'victims', 'volunteers' and 'experts', in CARTER, E. and WATNEY, S. (Eds) *Taking Liberties: AIDS and Cultural Politics*, pp. 113–25, London: Serpent's Tail.

PATTON, C., 1990, *Inventing AIDS*, London: Routledge.

PENNY, R., 1988, Changing perspectives 1982–1988, *Report of the Third National Conference on AIDS, Living with AIDS, Toward the Year 2000*, Hobart, 4–6 August 1988, Department of Community Services and Health, pp. 76–8, Canberra: Australian Government Printing Service.

PHILO, G., 1983, Bias in the media, in COATES, D. and JOHNSTON, G. (Eds) *Socialist Arguments*, pp. 130–45, Oxford: Martin Robertson.

POIRIER, R., 1988, AIDS and traditions of homophobia, *Social Research*, **55**, 3, 461–75.

POTTER, J. and WETHERELL, M., 1987, *Discourse and Social Psychology: Beyond Attitudes and Behaviour*, London: Sage.

POTTER, J., WETHERELL, M. and CHITTY, A., 1991, Quantification rhetoric – cancer on television, *Discourse and Society*, **2**, 3, 333–65.

REDMAN, R., 1991, Invasion of the monstrous others: identity, genre and HIV, *Cultural Studies from Birmingham*, **1**, 8–28.

REID, E., 1988, National strategy in Australia, *Report of the Third National Conference on AIDS, Living with AIDS, Toward the Year 2000*, Hobart, 4–6 August 1988. Department of Community Services and Health, pp. 106–12, Canberra: Australian Government Printing Service.

RHODES, T. and SHAUGHNESSY, R., 1990, Compulsory screening: advertising AIDS in Britain, 1986–89, *Policy and Politics*, **18**, 1, 55–61.

ROEH, I. and FELDMAN, S., 1984, The rhetoric of numbers in front-page journalism: how numbers contribute to the melodramatic in the popular press, *Text*, **4**, 4, 347–68.

ROGERS, E.M., DEARING, J.W. and CHANG, S., 1991, AIDS in the 1980s: the agenda-setting process for a public issue, *Journalism Monographs No. 126*, Columbia, South Carolina: Association for Education in Journalism and Mass Communication.

ROSENBERG, C.E., 1986, Disease and social order in America: perceptions and expectations, *Milbank Memorial Quarterly*, **64**, supp. 1, 34–55.

ROSS, J.W., 1989, An ethics of compassion, a language of division:

working out the AIDS metaphors, in CORLESS, I.B. and PITTMAN-LINDEMAN, M. (Eds) *AIDS: Principles, Practices and Politics*, pp. 351–63, NY: Hemisphere.

ROSS, M.W. and CARSON, J.A., 1988, Effectiveness of distribution of information on AIDS: a national study of six media in Australia, *New York State Journal of Medicine*, 239–41.

ROSS, M.W., 1989, Psychosocial ethical aspects of AIDS, *Journal of Medical Ethics*, **15**, 74–81.

RYAN, M., DUNWOODY, S. and TANKARD, J., 1991, Risk information for public consumption: print media coverage of two risky situations, *Health Education Quarterly*, **18**, 3, 375–90.

SCHUDSON, M., 1989, The sociology of news production, *Media, Culture and Society*, **11**, 263–82.

SEARS, A., 1992, 'To teach them how to live': the politics of public health from tuberculosis to AIDS, *Journal of Historical Sociology*, **5**, 1, 61–83.

SEIDMAN, S., 1991, *Romantic Longings: Love in America, 1830–1980*, NY: Routledge.

SEIDMAN, S., 1992, *Embattled Eros: Sexual Politics and Ethics in Contemporary America*, NY: Routledge.

SHEPHERD, R.G., 1981, Selectivity of sources; reporting the marijuana controversy, *Journal of Communication*, **31**, 2, 129–37.

SHOWALTER, E., 1990, *Sexual Anarchy: Gender and Culture at the Fin de Siècle*, NY: Viking.

SINGER, L., 1993, *Erotic Welfare: Sexual Theory and Politics in the Age of Epidemic*, NY: Routledge.

SONTAG, S., 1989, *Illness as Metaphor/AIDS and Its Metaphors*, NY: Anchor.

STREET, J. and WEALE, A., 1992, Britain, policy-making in a hermetically sealed system, in KIRP, D.L. and BAYER, R. (Eds) *AIDS in the Industrialized Democracies: Passions, Politics, and Policies*, pp. 185–220, New Brunswick: Rutgers University Press.

STRONG, P., 1990, Epidemic psychology: a model, *Sociology of Health and Illness*, **12**, 3, 249–59.

TEMOSHOK, L., GRADE, M. and ZICH, J., 1989, Public health, the press, and AIDS: an analysis of newspaper articles in London and San Francisco, in CORLESS, I.B. and PITTMAN-LINDEMAN, M. (Eds) *AIDS: Principles, Practices, and Politics.* pp. 535–52, NY: Hemisphere.

TREICHLER, P.A., 1988, AIDS, gender and biomedical discourse: current contests for meaning, in FEE, E., and FOX, D.M., (Eds) *AIDS: the Burdens of History*, pp. 190–266, Berkeley: University of California Press.

TREICHLER, P.A., 1980, AIDS, homophobia, and biomedical discourse:

an epidemic of signification, in CRIMP, D. (Ed.) *AIDS: Cultural Analysis, Cultural Activism,* pp. 31–70, Cambridge, Massachussetts: MIT Press.

TREICHLER, P.A., 1991, How to have theory in an epidemic: the evolution of AIDS treatment activism, in ROSS, A. and PENLEY, C., (Eds) *Technoculture,* pp. 57–106, Minneapolis: University of Minnesota Press.

TUCHMAN, G., 1978, *Making News: A Study in the Construction of Reality,* NY: Free Press.

TUCKEY, W., 1988, The politics of AIDS, *Report of the Third National Conference on AIDS, Living with AIDS, Toward the Year 2000,* Hobart, 4–6 August 1988. Department of Community Services and Health, pp. 739–41, Canberra: Australian Government Printing Service.

TULLOCH, J., 1989, Australian television and the representation of AIDS, *Australian Journal of Communication,* **16**, 101–24.

TULLOCH, J., 1992, Using TV in HIV/AIDS education: production and audience cultures, *Media Information Australia,* **65**, 28–35.

TURNER, B.A., 1984, *The Body and Society,* NY: Basil Blackwell.

VAN DIJK, T.A., 1984, *Prejudice in Discourse,* Amsterdam: John Benjamins.

VAN DIJK, T.A., 1991, *Racism and the Press,* London: Routledge.

WALDBY, C., KIPPAX, S. and CRAWFORD, J., 1991, Equality and eroticism: AIDS and the active/passive distinction, *Social Semiotics,* **1,** 2, 39–50.

WARWICK, I., AGGLETON, P. and HOMANS, H., 1988, Constructing commonsense – young people's beliefs about AIDS, *Sociology of Health and Illness,* **10**, 3, 213–33.

WATERSON, A., 1983, Acquired immune deficiency syndrome, *British Medical Journal,* **286**, 743–6.

WATNEY, S., 1987, *Policing Desire: Pornography, AIDS and the Media,* London: Comedia.

WATNEY, S., 1989a, The subject of AIDS, in AGGLETON, P., HART, G. and DAVIES, P. (Eds) *AIDS: Social Representations, Social Practices,* pp. 64–73, Basingstoke: Falmer.

WATNEY, S., 1989b, The spectacle of AIDS, in CRIMP, D. (Ed.) *AIDS: Cultural Analysis, Cultural Activism,* pp. 71–86, Cambridge, Massachusetts: MIT Press.

WATNEY, S., 1989c, Taking liberties: an introduction, in CARTER, E. and WATNEY, S. (Eds) *Taking Liberties,* pp. 11–57, London: Serpent's Tail.

WEBER, J. and GOLDMEIER, D., 1983, Medicine and the media, *British Medical Journal,* **287**, 420.

WEEKS, J., 1986, *Sexuality,* London: Tavistock.

WEEKS, J., 1989, AIDS: the intellectual agenda, in AGGLETON, P., HART, G., and DAVIES, P. (Eds) *AIDS: Social Representations, Social Practices*, pp. 1–20, Basingstoke: Falmer.

WELLINGS, K., 1988, Perceptions of risk – media treatment of AIDS, in AGGLETON, P., and HOMANS, H. (Eds) *Social Aspects of AIDS*, pp. 83–105, Basingstoke: Falmer.

WHITE, D.G., PHILLIPS, K.C., PITTS, M., *et al.*, 1988, Adolescents' perceptions of AIDS, *Health Education Journal*, **47**, 4, 117–27.

WILLIAMSON, J., 1989, Every virus tells a story, in CARTER, E. and WATNEY, S. (Eds) *Taking Liberties*, pp. 69–80, London: Serpent's Tail.

WILTON, T. and AGGLETON, P., 1991, Condoms, coercion and control: heterosexuality and the limits to HIV/AIDS education, in AGGLETON, P., HART, G. and DAVIES, P. (Eds) *AIDS: Responses, Interventions and Care*, pp. 149–56, London: Falmer.

WORLD HEALTH ORGANIZATION, 1986, *Ottawa Charter for Health Promotion: Report of the International Conference on Health Promotion* 17–21 November 1986, Ottawa, World Health Organization.

WRIGHT, P. and TREACHER, A., 1982, Introduction, in WRIGHT, P. and TREACHER, A. (Eds) *The Problem of Medical Knowledge: Examining the Social Construction of Medicine*, pp. 1–22, Edinburgh: Edinburgh University Press.

YOUNG, J., 1981, Beyond the consensual paradigm: a critique of left functionalism in media theory, in COHEN, S. and YOUNG, J. (Eds) *The Manufacture of News: Social Problems, Deviance and the Mass Media* (revised), pp. 393–421, London: Constable.

Index